The Complete

Low Cholesterol

Cookbook for Beginners

1800 Days of Delightful & Easy Recipes to Keep Your Heart Healthy and Eat Well |Stress-Free 30-Day Meal Plan to Lower Cholesterol

Barbara F. Gibson

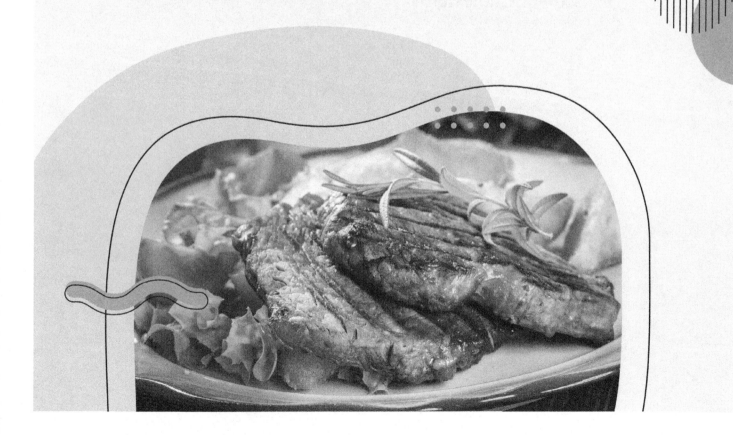

Savor the healthy changes of a low cholesterol diet together!

Get a primer on low cholesterol and arm yourself with knowledge

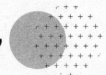

Every bite of food you eat is heart-healthy

Each recipe is made with care and is beginner-friendly

Reduce preparation time by using ingredients that are readily available at local markets

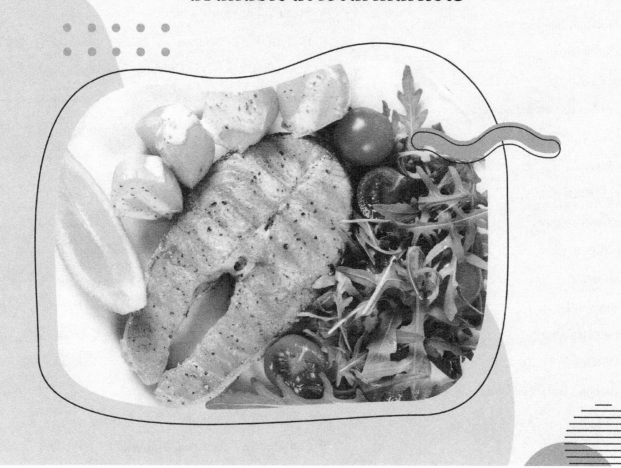

CONTENTS

Sauces, Dressings, And Staples... 76

Desserts And Treats 84

30–Day Meal Plan 94

Measurement Conversions.......... 96

Shopping Lists 98

Appendix : Recipes Index............ 101

INTRODUCTION

I'm Barbara F. Gibson, a culinary writer with a wealth of experience and passion. Throughout my career, I have been dedicated to combining good food with healthy living, hoping that through my recipes, I can help people enjoy good food and maintain a healthy lifestyle at the same time.

In the process, I realized that many people are increasingly passionate about cooking and staying healthy, but know little about how to eat a cholesterol-lowering diet. This led me to decide to write a recipe book called The Low Cholesterol Cookbook. The goal of this book is to help people who need to lower their cholesterol by providing practical cooking tips and healthy recipes that they can enjoy while staying healthy.

In this book, I provide readers with detailed step-by-step instructions so that everyone can easily master every aspect of cooking. Whether you are a beginner or someone with some basic cooking skills, you will be able to find the right cooking tips for you in this book. In addition, the book also contains some bonus DIY and shopping lists to help you buy ingredients more conveniently.

Each dish is labeled with cooking time, so you can keep better track of the cooking progress. I've also shared a list of useful cooking tips to help you get the most out of your cooking. These tips include how to choose healthy ingredients, how to control oil and salt intake, and how to mix and match ingredients.

I hope that through this book, more people will understand the importance of a low cholesterol diet, and that it will provide practical cooking guidelines for those who need to lower their cholesterol. I believe that if you are willing to give it a try, you will be able to enjoy good food and live a healthy life at the same time.

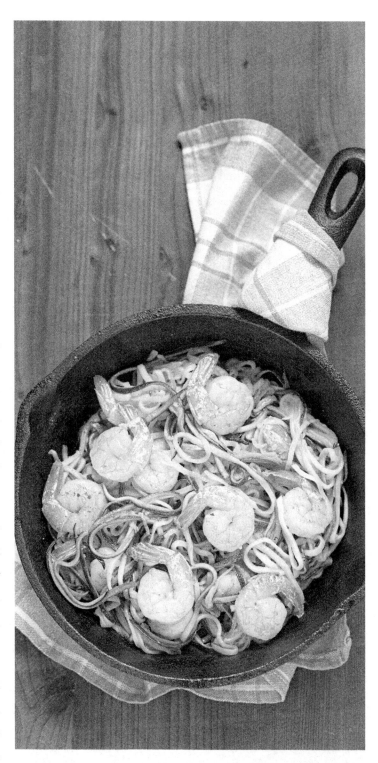

What is Low Cholesterol?

Low cholesterol typically means having lower levels of cholesterol in the blood, particularly low levels of LDL (low-density lipoprotein) cholesterol. This is generally considered beneficial for heart health as it reduces the risk of atherosclerosis and related cardiovascular problems. However, extremely low cholesterol levels can sometimes raise health concerns due to the essential role of cholesterol in various bodily functions.

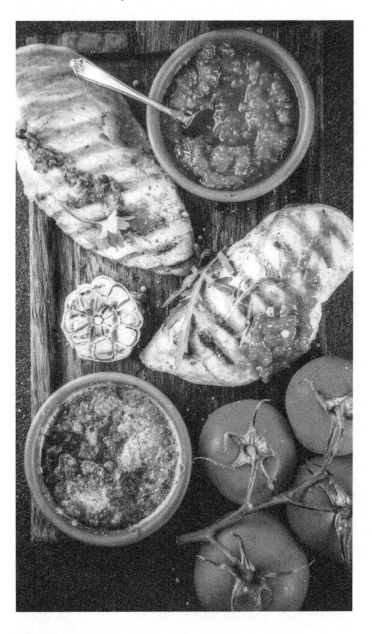

What are the common Low Cholesterol foods?

Fruits and Vegetables: High fiber, low cholesterol.

Whole Grains: Fiber-rich, reduce LDL.

Legumes: Plant-based protein, heart-healthy.

Nuts and Seeds: Healthy fats, lower cholesterol.

Fatty Fish: Omega-3, reduces risk.

Skinless Poultry: Lean protein, less saturated fat.

Low-Fat Dairy: Essential nutrients, lower fat.

Plant-Based Oils: Heart-healthy cooking.

Herbs and Spices: Flavor without salt.

Avocado: Nutrient-rich, healthy fats.

Tofu and Soy: Low saturated fat.

Egg Whites: Low-cholesterol alternative.

What do people with high cholesterol need to pay attention to in their lives?

Diet: Adopt a heart-healthy diet. Focus on reducing saturated fats, trans fats, and dietary cholesterol. Emphasize fruits, vegetables, whole grains, lean proteins, and foods rich in soluble fiber.

Portion Control: Be mindful of portion sizes to avoid overeating, which can lead to excess calorie and fat intake.

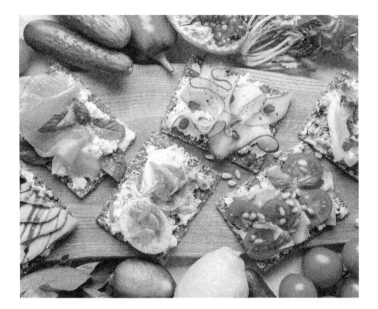

Label Reading: Read food labels to identify and limit products high in saturated and trans fats. Pay attention to cholesterol content in foods.

Regular Exercise: Engage in regular physical activity. Aim for at least 150 minutes of moderate-intensity aerobic exercise or 75 minutes of vigorous exercise per week, along with strength training.

Weight Management: Maintain a healthy weight or lose excess weight if necessary. Weight loss can improve cholesterol levels.

What benefits can this Low Cholesterol Cookbook bring?

HEART HEALTH IMPROVEMENT:

- A Low Cholesterol Cookbook provides recipes specifically designed to reduce cholesterol levels. By following these recipes, you can actively work to lower LDL (bad) cholesterol and triglycerides, promoting better heart health and reducing the risk of heart disease.

LOWER RISK OF HEART DISEASE:

- High cholesterol is a significant risk factor for heart disease. A low cholesterol diet, facilitated by the cookbook, can help lower this risk by reducing the accumulation of plaque in the arteries, which can lead to heart attacks and strokes.

WEIGHT MANAGEMENT:

- Many low cholesterol recipes also tend to be low in saturated fats and processed sugars. By using these recipes, you can manage your weight more effectively, reducing the risk of obesity-related health issues.

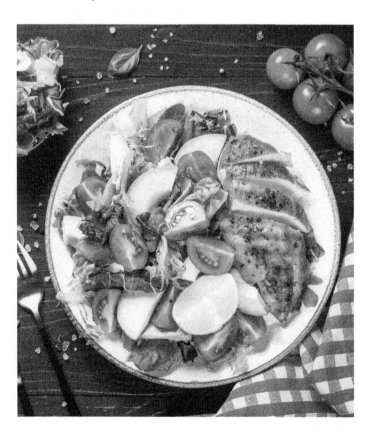

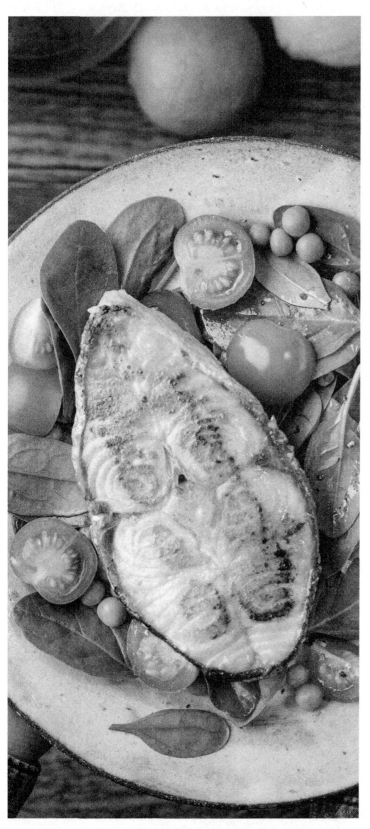

BALANCED NUTRITION:

- A well-constructed cookbook offers recipes that not only help lower cholesterol but also ensure balanced nutrition. This means you'll receive essential nutrients, promoting overall well-being.

VARIETY AND FLAVOR:

- Low cholesterol recipes are not limited to bland or unappetizing options. A high-quality cookbook provides a wide range of delicious and satisfying meals that make it easier to adhere to a low cholesterol diet without feeling deprived.

FAMILY-FRIENDLY:

- These cookbooks offer recipes that are suitable for the entire family, which simplifies meal preparation and ensures that everyone in the household can enjoy heart-healthy meals together.

PORTION CONTROL:

- Portion control is an important aspect of managing cholesterol and overall calorie intake. Many low cholesterol cookbooks provide portion recommendations to help you maintain a healthy weight.

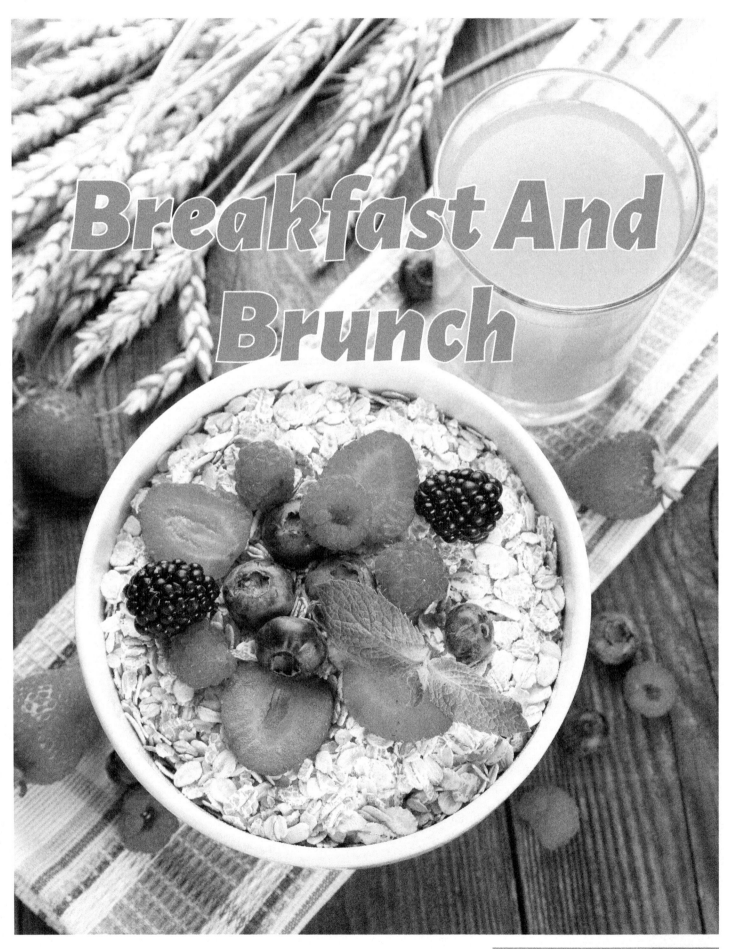

Breakfast And Brunch

Breakfast And Brunch

Panzanella Breakfast Casserole

Servings: X

Cooking Time: 35 Minutes

Ingredients:

- Nonstick olive oil cooking spray
- 1 teaspoon olive oil
- ¼ cup chopped sweet onion
- 1 teaspoon minced garlic
- 2 slices multigrain bread, cut into ½-inch chunks
- ¼ cup chopped artichoke hearts
- ¼ cup sliced black olives
- ¼ cup sliced sun-dried tomatoes
- 12 ounces firm tofu, drained and pressed (see tip, Chili-Sautéed Tofu with Almonds)
- ½ cup soy milk
- ½ teaspoon chopped fresh basil

Directions:

1. Preheat the oven to 350°F. Lightly spray 2 (8-ounce) ramekins with cooking spray and set aside.
2. Warm the olive oil in a small skillet over medium-high heat.
3. Add the onion and garlic and sauté until translucent, about 3 minutes.
4. Transfer the onion mixture to a medium bowl and stir in the bread, artichoke hearts, olives, and sun-dried tomatoes, tossing well to mix.
5. In a blender, add the tofu and soy milk and blend until smooth.
6. Add the tofu mixture to the bowl with the bread, add the basil, and stir to combine.
7. Evenly divide the mixture between the ramekins, shaking them to evenly disperse the mixture.
8. Place the ramekins on a baking sheet and bake until the casseroles are set and golden brown, 25 to 30 minutes.
9. Serve.

Nutrition Info:

- Per Serving: Calories: 294 ; Fat: 13 g ;Saturated fat: 2 g ;Sodium: 147 mg

Pineapple Mixed Berry Smoothie

Servings: 2

Cooking Time: X

Ingredients:

- 1 cup sliced strawberries
- ½ cup raspberries
- ½ cup cubed pineapple
- ½ cup low-fat soy milk
- 1 tablespoon fresh lemon juice
- 1 scoop protein powder
- 1 cup ice cubes

Directions:

1. In a blender or food processor, combine the strawberries, raspberries, pineapple, soy milk, lemon juice, and protein powder.
2. Cover and blend until almost smooth.
3. Add the ice, cover, and blend until the mixture is thick and smooth. Pour into 2 tall glasses. Serve immediately.

Nutrition Info:

- Per Serving: Calories: 138; Fat: 2 g ;Saturated fat: 0 g ;Sodium: 163 mg

Blueberry Smoothie Bowl

Servings: 2

Cooking Time: 10 Minutes

Ingredients:

- 1 cup fresh berries (such as strawberries, blueberries, or blackberries), plus more for topping
- 1 banana
- ½ cup low-fat plain Greek yogurt
- ½ cup low-fat milk
- 1 tablespoon crushed almonds

Directions:

1. In a blender, place the berries, banana, yogurt, and milk and blend until smooth.
2. Pour the smoothie into a bowl and top with crushed almonds and fresh berries.

Nutrition Info:

- Per Serving: Calories: 140; Fat :2g ;Saturated fat: 0g;Sodium: 56mg

Pb&j Smoothies

Servings: 3

Cooking Time: X

Ingredients:

- 1 cup raspberry yogurt
- 1 cup skim milk
- 3 tablespoons peanut butter
- ½ cup frozen vanilla yogurt
- 2 tablespoons raspberry jelly

Directions:

1. In blender or food processor, combine yogurt, milk, peanut butter, and frozen yogurt. Blend or process until smooth. By hand, stir in the jelly just until marbled.

Pour into glasses and serve immediately.

Nutrition Info:

- Per Serving: Calories: 238.61 ; Fat: 9.89 g ;Saturated fat:2.47 g ;Sodium: 92.47 mg

Fish Tacos

Servings: 5

Cooking Time: 20 Minutes

Ingredients:

- 1 pound white fish (such as tilapia), cut into bite-size pieces
- 1 tablespoon olive oil
- Sea salt
- Freshly ground black pepper
- 1 cup low-fat plain Greek yogurt
- 5 (6½-inch) whole wheat or whole-grain corn tortillas
- 2½ cups shredded romaine lettuce
- 2 tablespoons freshly squeezed lime juice

Directions:

1. In a medium bowl, mix the salmon, Spicy Honey Sauce, and Preheat the oven to 375°F. Line a baking sheet with parchment paper.
2. Season the fish with the olive oil, salt, and pepper. Place the fish on the prepared baking sheet and bake for 20 minutes, until slightly golden brown.
3. While the fish is cooking, in a small bowl, combine the yogurt with another pinch of salt and pepper.
4. Once the fish is cooked, place ⅕ of the fish in a tortilla with ½ cup romaine, 1 teaspoon lime juice, and a dollop of yogurt. Repeat with the remaining tortillas and serve immediately.

Nutrition Info:

- Per Serving: Calories: 272; Fat: 7g ;Saturated fat: 2g ;Sodium: 450mg

Light Whole-grain Bread

Servings: 32

Cooking Time: X

Ingredients:

- 1 cup lukewarm water
- 2 (¼-ounce) packages active dry yeast
- 1½ cups buttermilk
- ½ cup orange juice
- ½ teaspoon salt
- 1/3 cup honey
- 3 tablespoons canola oil
- 1 egg
- 2 cups whole-wheat flour
- ½ cup oat bran
- ½ cup cracked wheat
- 3½ to 4½ cups bread flour
- ½ teaspoon baking soda
- 2 tablespoons butter

Directions:

1. In large bowl, combine water and yeast; mix well and let stand for 10 minutes. Add buttermilk, orange juice, salt, honey, oil, and egg and beat well. Add 1 cup whole-wheat flour, oat bran, cracked wheat, 1 cup bread flour, and baking soda; beat for 1 minute. Let bread stand for 30 minutes.
2. Gradually add enough remaining whole-wheat flour and bread flour to form a firm dough. Turn onto floured surface and knead for 10 minutes. Place dough in greased bowl, turning to grease top. Cover and let rise for 1 hour.
3. Turn dough onto floured work surface and let rest for 10 minutes. Grease two 9″ × 5″ loaf pans with unsalted butter and set aside. Punch down dough and divide into two parts. On floured surface, roll or pat to 7″ × 12″ rectangle. Roll up tightly, starting with 7″ side. Place in prepared pans.
4. Cover with towel, and let rise until double, about 30 minutes. Preheat oven to 350ºF. Bake loaves for 35–45 minutes or until golden brown. Brush each loaf with butter, then turn onto wire rack to cool completely.

Nutrition Info:

- Per Serving: Calories:137.87; Fat: 2.75 g ;Saturated fat:0.74g ;Sodium: 76.58 mg

Cogrilled Meatloaf Sandwiches

Servings: 6–8

Cooking Time: X

Ingredients:

- 2 tablespoons ketchup
- 2 tablespoons mustard
- 2 tablespoons grated Parmesan cheese
- 4 slices Whole-Grain Meatloaf , cooked and chilled
- 8 slices Whole-Grain Oatmeal Bread
- 1 tomato, thinly sliced
- ½ cup shredded extra-sharp Cheddar cheese
- 2 tablespoons olive oil

Directions:

1. Preheat indoor dual-contact grill or griddle. In small bowl, combine ketchup, mustard, and Parmesan cheese. Spread on both sides of the meatloaf; place one slice of meatloaf on one slice of bread.
2. Top with tomato slices, then Cheddar cheese. Top with rest of bread slices. Brush outsides of sandwiches with olive oil. Grill sandwiches on dual-contact grill for 3–4 minutes each, or grill on a griddle, turning once, for 6–9 minutes until bread is golden brown and meatloaf is hot. Cut in half and serve immediately.

Nutrition Info:

- Per Serving: Calories:364.06 ; Fat: 16.35 g ;Saturated fat:5.47 g ;Sodium: 326.11 mg

Zucchini-walnut Bread

Servings: 12

Cooking Time: X

Ingredients:

- ¼ cup canola oil
- ¼ cup sugar
- ½ cup brown sugar
- 1 egg
- 2 egg whites
- ½ cup orange juice
- 2 teaspoons vanilla
- 1 cup grated zucchini
- 1 teaspoon grated lemon zest
- 2 tablespoons wheat germ
- 1 cup all-purpose flour
- 1 cup whole-wheat flour
- 1 teaspoon baking powder
- ½ teaspoon baking soda
- 1/8 teaspoon salt
- 1 teaspoon cinnamon
- ¼ teaspoon cloves
- ½ cup chopped walnuts

Directions:

1. Preheat oven to 350ºF. Spray a 9″ × 5″ loaf pan with nonstick cooking spray containing flour, and set aside.
2. In large bowl, combine oil, sugar, brown sugar, egg, egg whites, orange juice, and vanilla and beat until smooth. Stir in zucchini, lemon zest, and wheat germ.
3. Sift together flour, whole-wheat flour, baking powder, baking soda, salt, cinnamon, and cloves, and add to oil mixture. Stir just until combined, then fold in walnuts. Pour into prepared pan.
4. Bake for 55–65 minutes or until bread is golden-brown and toothpick inserted in center comes out clean. Remove from pan and let cool on wire rack.

Nutrition Info:

- Per Serving: Calories:217.46 ; Fat: 8.48 g ;Saturated fat:0.70 g;Sodium: 127.63 mg

Dutch Baby Pancakes

Servings: X

Cooking Time: 25 Minutes

Ingredients:

- 2 large egg whites
- ¼ cup almond flour
- ¼ cup all-purpose flour
- ½ cup unsweetened soy milk
- 1 teaspoon granulated sugar
- 1 teaspoon pure vanilla extract
- ⅛ teaspoon ground nutmeg
- Pinch sea salt
- Butter-flavored nonstick cooking spray, for greasing the pan
- 1 teaspoon canola oil

Directions:

1. Preheat the oven to 425°F.
2. In a medium bowl, whisk the egg whites, almond flour, all-purpose flour, soy milk, sugar, vanilla, nutmeg, and salt until well blended into a batter.
3. Spray a medium skillet (cast iron, preferably) with cooking spray and add the oil, tilting the skillet to coat the bottom. Place the skillet in the oven for 10 minutes to let it heat up.
4. Remove the skillet from the oven and pour in the batter. Return the skillet to the oven and bake the pancake until it is golden brown and puffed, about 15 minutes.
5. Remove from the oven and serve hot.

Nutrition Info:

- Per Serving: Calories: 176 ; Fat: 7 g ;Saturated fat: 1 g ;Sodium: 167 mg

Honey-wheat Sesame Bread

Servings: 32

Cooking Time: X

Ingredients:

- 1 cup milk
- 1 cup water
- ½ cup honey
- 3 tablespoons butter
- ¼ teaspoon salt
- 1 egg
- 2 cups whole-wheat flour
- 2 (¼-ounce) packages instant-blend dry yeast
- ½ cup sesame seeds
- 3 to 4 cups all-purpose flour
- 1 egg white
- 2 tablespoons sesame seeds

Directions:

1. In medium saucepan, combine milk, water, honey, butter, and salt. Heat over medium heat until butter melts. Remove from heat and let stand for 30 minutes or until just lukewarm. Beat in egg.
2. Meanwhile, in large bowl combine whole-wheat flour, instant-blend yeast, and ½ cup sesame seeds. Add milk mixture and beat for 1 minute. Then gradually stir in enough all-purpose flour to make a firm dough.
3. Turn out onto floured surface and knead, adding additional flour if necessary, until dough is elastic. Place in greased bowl, turning to grease top; cover and let rise until double, about 1 hour.
4. Grease two 9″ × 5″ loaf pans with unsalted butter and set aside. Punch down dough and divide into two parts. On floured surface, roll or pat to 7″ × 12″ rectangle. Roll up tightly, starting with 7″ side. Place in prepared pans. Brush with egg white and sprinkle each with 1 tablespoon sesame seeds.
5. Cover with towel, and let rise until double, about 30 minutes. Preheat oven to 350ºF. Bake loaves for 35–45 minutes or until golden brown. Turn onto wire rack to cool completely.

Nutrition Info:

- Per Serving: Calories: 131.38; Fat: 3.02 g ;Saturated fat: 1.03 g ;Sodium: 34.51 mg

Tofu Scramble With Tomato And Spinach

Servings: X

Cooking Time: 15 Minutes

Ingredients:

- 2 teaspoons olive oil
- ¼ cup chopped sweet onion
- 1 cup halved cherry tomatoes
- 1 cup fresh baby spinach
- 10 ounces firm tofu, crumbled into small pieces
- ¼ cup low-fat cottage cheese
- 1 teaspoon chopped fresh oregano
- Sea salt
- Freshly ground black pepper

Directions:

1. Warm the olive oil in a medium nonstick skillet over medium heat.
2. Add the onion to the pan and sauté until translucent, about 3 minutes.
3. Add the tomatoes and spinach and sauté until the spinach is wilted, about 3 minutes.
4. Add the tofu to the skillet and gently stir using a rubber spatula until warmed through, about 7 minutes.
5. Fold in the cottage cheese and oregano.
6. Season with salt and pepper and serve.

Nutrition Info:

- Per Serving: Calories: 201 ; Fat: 5 g ;Saturated fat: 1 g ;Sodium: 97 mg

Nutty Oat Bars

Servings: 6

Cooking Time: 7 Minutes

Ingredients:

- Olive oil
- 1 cup pitted Medjool dates
- 1 cup steel-cut oats
- ½ cup nut butter (such as almond, cashew, or all-natural peanut butter)
- 2 tablespoons maple syrup
- ½ cup almonds

Directions:

1. Lightly coat a 4-by-8-inch baking pan with olive oil.
2. In a blender or food processor, process the dates until a paste forms, about 2 minutes.
3. Place the oats in a medium skillet over low heat and toast for 5 minutes or until the edges turn brown. Set aside.
4. In a medium saucepan, combine the nut butter and maple syrup over medium heat, and cook for 1 to 2 minutes, stirring with a wooden spoon.
5. In a medium bowl, mix the date paste, oats, nut butter mixture, and almonds until everything is coated well.
6. Press the oat mixture into the prepared baking pan and place it in the freezer until it sets, about 20 minutes.
7. Once set, cut into six bars and serve.

Nutrition Info:

- Per Serving: Calories:379; Fat: 19g ;Saturated fat: 1g ;Sodium: 3mg

Seaweed Rice Rolls

Servings: 2

Cooking Time: X

Ingredients:

- ¾ cup short-grain brown rice, rinsed
- 1½ cups water
- 1 (4-ounce) can low-sodium tuna packed in water, drained
- ½ tablespoon sesame oil
- Sea salt
- Freshly ground black pepper
- 2 (7-by-8-inch) sheets dried seaweed
- 2 cups Sesame Spinach

Directions:

1. In a medium saucepan over high heat, combine the rice and the water and bring to a boil. Cover, reduce the heat to low, and simmer until the liquid is absorbed, about 30 minutes. Remove from the heat, fluff with a fork, and let cool.
2. In a small bowl, mix the tuna and sesame oil, and season with salt and pepper.
3. Place the seaweed sheets on a flat surface and evenly spread ¾ cup of the rice on one sheet.
4. Place half the tuna mixture and half the Sesame Spinach on the rice along one end of the seaweed.
5. Slowly roll up the seaweed rice wrap, starting at the end with the tuna and spinach, and gently press down to make a firm roll. Make sure to apply firm, even pressure over the entire roll when rolling.
6. Wet the end of the seaweed wrap with water to seal the roll. Repeat to make the other roll.
7. Cut the rolls into equal slices and enjoy immediately.

Nutrition Info:

- Per Serving: Calories: 481 ; Fat: 14g ;Saturated fat: 3g ;Sodium: 498mg

Spinach Artichoke Pizza

Servings: 8

Cooking Time: X

Ingredients:

- 1 (10-ounce) package frozen chopped spinach, thawed and drained
- 1 (9-ounce) package frozen artichoke hearts, thawed and drained
- 1 tablespoon olive oil
- 1 onion, chopped
- 3 cloves garlic, minced
- 1 red bell pepper, chopped
- 1 (8-ounce) package sliced mushrooms
- 1 cup part-skim ricotta cheese
- ¼ cup grated Parmesan cheese
- 1 cup shredded part-skim mozzarella cheese
- ½ cup shredded extra-sharp Cheddar cheese
- 1 Whole-Grain Pizza Crust

Directions:

1. Preheat oven to 400°F. Press spinach between paper towels to remove all excess moisture. Cut artichoke hearts into small pieces.
2. In large saucepan, heat olive oil. Cook onion, garlic, red pepper, and mushrooms until crisp-tender, about 4 minutes. Add spinach; cook and stir until liquid evaporates, about 5 minutes longer. Add mushrooms; cook and stir for 2–3 minutes longer.
3. Drain vegetable mixture if necessary. Place in medium bowl and let cool for 20 minutes. Then blend in ricotta and Parmesan cheeses.
4. Spread on pizza crust. Top with mozzarella and Cheddar cheeses. Bake for 20–25 minutes or until pizza is hot and cheese is melted and begins to brown. Serve immediately.

Nutrition Info:

- Per Serving: Calories: 335.56; Fat:13.05 g ;Saturated fat: 6.06 g ;Sodium: 317.04 mg

Strawberry Yogurt Tarts

Servings: 5

Cooking Time: 2 Hours

Ingredients:

- ½ cup pitted Medjool dates
- ½ cup crushed almonds
- 1 tablespoon maple syrup
- 1 cup low-fat plain Greek yogurt
- ½ cup strawberries
- 2 tablespoons water

Directions:

1. Line 5 cups of a muffin tin with paper liners and set aside.
2. In a food processor or blender, place the dates and pulse for 10 to 20 seconds until they become a paste.
3. Add the crushed almonds and maple syrup to the blender and pulse to mix.
4. Evenly divide the date mixture into the lined cups and press it down firmly; it should fill about one-third of the cup.
5. In a clean blender, blend the yogurt, strawberries, and water until smooth.
6. Pour the fruit and yogurt mixture into the cups until each one is full.
7. Place the cups in the freezer for 2 hours to set, and serve.

Nutrition Info:

- Per Serving: Calories: 141; Fat:5g ;Saturated fat:1g ;Sodium: 35mg

Navajo Chili Bread

Servings: 12

Cooking Time: X

Ingredients:

- 3 tablespoons olive oil
- ½ cup minced onion
- 2 cloves garlic, minced
- 2 jalapeño peppers, minced
- ½ cup finely chopped red bell pepper
- 1¼ cups all-purpose flour
- 1 cup yellow cornmeal
- 1/8 teaspoon salt
- 1 teaspoon baking powder
- ½ teaspoon baking soda
- 2 teaspoons chili powder
- ½ cup liquid egg substitute
- ¼ cup buttermilk
- 2 tablespoons molasses
- ½ cup shredded Pepper Jack cheese

Directions:

1. Preheat oven to 375ºF. Spray a 9″ square glass baking dish with nonstick cooking spray containing flour, and set aside.
2. In small saucepan, heat olive oil over medium heat Add onion, garlic, jalapeño, and red bell pepper; cook and stir until crisp-tender, about 4 minutes. Remove from heat.
3. In large bowl, combine flour, cornmeal, salt, baking powder, baking soda, and chili powder, and mix to combine. Add egg substitute, buttermilk, and molasses to vegetables in saucepan, and beat to combine. Stir into flour mixture until combined, then fold in cheese.
4. Pour batter into prepared pan. Bake for 30–40 minutes or until bread is light golden-brown and toothpick inserted in center comes out clean. Let cool for 15 minutes, then serve.

Nutrition Info:

- Per Serving: Calories:223.97 ; Fat:7.59 g ;Saturated fat:2.11 g ;Sodium: 232.04 mg

Nutty Quinoa Waffles

Servings: 4

Cooking Time: 15 Minutes

Ingredients:

- 1 cup quinoa flour
- 1½ teaspoons baking powder
- 1 teaspoon ground cinnamon
- ⅛ teaspoon ground nutmeg
- Pinch salt
- 1 egg, separated
- ½ cup almond or soy milk
- 2 tablespoons honey or pure maple syrup
- 1 teaspoon vanilla extract
- 3 tablespoons ground pecans

Directions:

1. In a medium bowl, combine the quinoa flour, baking powder, cinnamon, nutmeg, and salt and blend well with a wire whisk or fork.
2. In a small bowl, combine the egg yolk, almond milk, honey, and vanilla and mix well.
3. In another medium bowl, beat the egg white until stiff.
4. Stir the egg yolk mixture into the dry ingredients, then fold in the egg white.
5. Preheat a waffle iron and spray it with nonstick cooking spray.
6. Add batter to the waffle iron per the manufacturer's instructions. Close the iron and cook until the steaming stops, 4 to 5 minutes. Remove the waffle from the iron, sprinkle with ground pecans, and serve immediately.

Nutrition Info:

- Per Serving: Calories: 195 ; Fat: 7 g ;Saturated fat: 1 g ;Sodium: 169 mg

Chicken Pesto Baguette

Servings: 6

Cooking Time: 20 Minutes

Ingredients:

- 1 pound boneless, skinless chicken breast
- 5 cups water
- 1 cup low-fat plain Greek yogurt
- 1½ cups Spinach and Walnut Pesto
- 2½ cups arugula
- 2 (12-inch) whole wheat or whole-grain baguettes, halved lengthwise

Directions:

1. In a large skillet, cover the chicken with the water and poach for 20 minutes over medium-high heat.
2. Remove the chicken from the water, let it cool, and finely dice the chicken.
3. In a large bowl, mix the diced chicken, yogurt, and Spinach and Walnut Pesto until combined.
4. Arrange the arugula on the baguettes and evenly divide the chicken salad between them. Slice each baguette into three equal parts. Serve immediately.

Nutrition Info:

- Per Serving: Calories: 527 ; Fat: 33 g ;Saturated fat: 5 g ;Sodium: 499 mg

Vegetable Omelet

Servings: 4

Cooking Time: X

Ingredients:

- 1 tablespoon olive oil
- ½ cup grated carrot
- ½ cup chopped broccoli
- ¼ cup finely chopped red onion
- 8 egg whites 1 egg yolk
- ¼ cup 1% milk
- 1/8 teaspoon white pepper

- ½ cup grated extra-sharp Cheddar cheese

Directions:

1. In large nonstick skillet, heat olive oil over medium heat. Add carrot, broccoli, and onion; cook, stirring occasionally, until crisp-tender, about 4–5 minutes.
2. Meanwhile, in medium bowl, beat egg whites until a soft foam forms. In small bowl, combine egg yolk with milk and pepper and beat well. Fold egg yolk mixture into egg whites.
3. Pour the egg mixture into the pan. Cook, lifting the edges of the eggs so the uncooked mixture can flow underneath, until eggs are set but still moist. Sprinkle with cheese and cover pan; cook for 1 minute. Uncover, fold omelet, and serve immediately.

Nutrition Info:

- Per Serving: Calories: 156.08; Fat: 9.54 g ;Saturated fat: 3.96 g;Sodium: 220.56 mg

Blueberry Almond Breakfast Bowl

Servings: 1

Cooking Time: 20 Minutes

Ingredients:

- ¾ cup full-fat plain Greek yogurt
- ⅔ cup blueberries, divided
- ½ small banana, cut into slices
- 1 tablespoon chia seeds
- 2 tablespoons low-fat almond milk
- 1 tablespoon sliced almonds, toasted

Directions:

1. In a blender or food processor, combine the yogurt, ¼ cup of the blueberries, the banana, chia seeds, and almond milk. Blend or process until smooth.
2. Spoon into a cereal bowl and top with the almonds and remaining blueberries.

Nutrition Info:

- Per Serving: Calories: 343 ; Fat: 15 g ;Saturated fat: 5 g ;Sodium: 109 mg

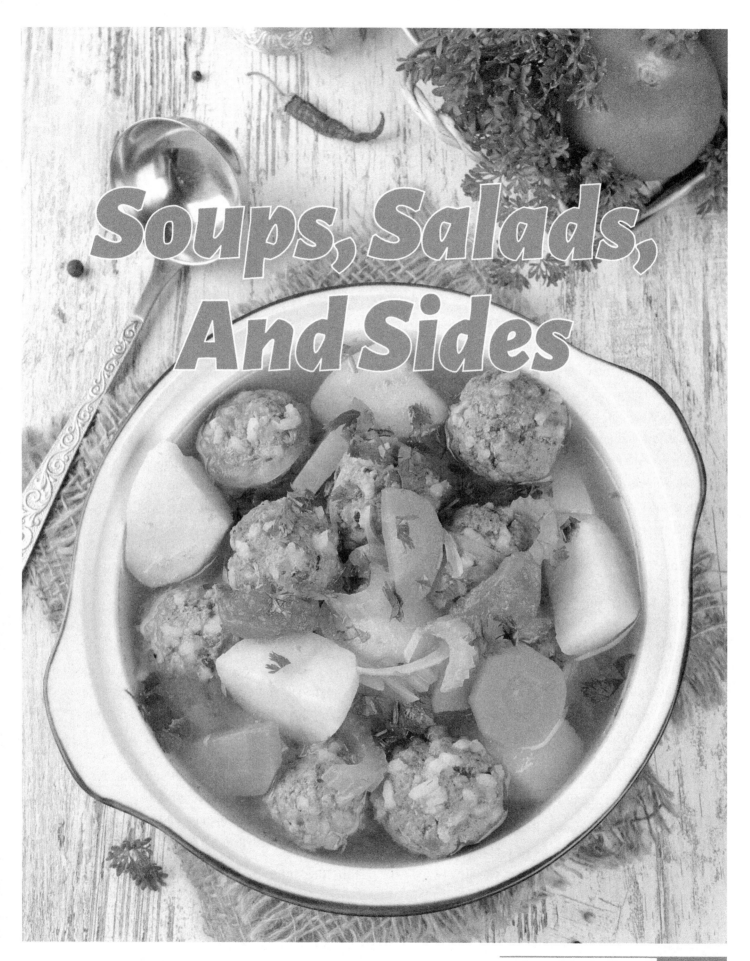

Soups, Salads, And Sides

Soups, Salads, And Sides

Thai Chicken Soup

Servings: 4

Cooking Time: 20 Minutes

Ingredients:

- 2 teaspoons olive oil
- 2 (6-ounce) boneless, skinless chicken breasts
- Pinch salt
- ⅛ teaspoon cayenne pepper
- 1 lemongrass stalk, peeled and chopped
- 4 cloves garlic, minced
- 1 jalapeño chile, seeded and minced
- 1 red bell pepper, seeded and chopped
- 2 cups low-sodium chicken stock
- 1 cup water
- 2 tablespoons fresh lime juice
- 1 teaspoon Thai chili paste
- ⅛ teaspoon ground ginger

Directions:

1. In a large saucepan, heat the olive oil over medium heat.
2. Sprinkle the chicken with the salt and cayenne pepper, and add it to the saucepan. Cook, turning once, until the chicken is browned, about 3 to 4 minutes per side. Transfer the chicken to a plate and set aside.
3. Add the lemongrass, garlic, jalapeño, and bell pepper to the saucepan, and cook for 3 minutes, stirring frequently.
4. Add the chicken stock and water to the saucepan, and stir and bring to a simmer. Return the chicken to the saucepan. Simmer for 10 to 12 minutes, or until the chicken is cooked to 165°F when tested with a meat thermometer.
5. Remove the chicken to a clean plate and shred, using two forks. Return the chicken to the soup.
6. Add the lime juice, chili paste, and ginger, and simmer for 2 minutes longer. Serve hot.

Nutrition Info:

- Per Serving: Calories: 134 ; Fat: 5 g ;Saturated fat: 1 g ;Sodium: 237 mg

Creamy Vegetable Soup

Servings: 4

Cooking Time: 40 Min

Ingredients:

- 1 tsp olive oil
- 1 medium red onion, finely chopped
- 2 medium carrots, peeled and diced
- 2 cups courgettes, diced
- 1 small red potato, peeled and diced
- 1 cup dried green split peas
- 4 cups low-sodium vegetable stock
- ¼ tsp ground black pepper

Directions:

1. In a large stockpot, heat the olive oil over medium heat and add the onion and carrots. Cook for 5 minutes until the onions are translucent and the carrots are lightly browned.
2. Add the courgettes, red potato, split peas, vegetable stock, and pepper. Mix well and cook for 35 minutes on a low boil, partially covered.
3. Use an immersion blender and pulse 3 to 4 times until desired consistency. Serve hot.

Nutrition Info:

- Per Serving: Calories: 154; Fat: 2 g ;Saturated fat: 1 g ;Sodium: 178mg

Watermelon, Edamame, And Radish Salad

Servings: X

Cooking Time: X

Ingredients:

- 4 cups diced watermelon
- 2 cups shelled edamame
- 4 radishes, quartered
- 2 cups kale, torn into bite-size pieces
- ¼ cup Lemon-Cilantro Vinaigrette or store-bought balsamic vinaigrette
- ½ cup crumbled fat-free feta cheese, for garnish
- ¼ cup roasted, unsalted pumpkin seeds, for garnish

Directions:

1. In a medium bowl, add the watermelon, edamame, radishes, and kale.
2. Add the dressing and toss to coat.
3. Serve topped with feta and pumpkin seeds.

Nutrition Info:

- Per Serving: Calories: 514 ; Fat: 24 g ;Saturated fat: 3 g ;Sodium: 400 mg

Tangy Fish And Tofu Soup

Servings: 5

Cooking Time: 10 Minutes

Ingredients:

- 1 pound white fish (such as tilapia), thinly sliced
- ⅓ cup Tangy Soy Sauce
- 8 cups water
- 4 cups chopped napa cabbage
- 1 white onion, chopped
- 12 ounces soft tofu, cubed

Directions:

1. Place the fish and the Tangy Soy Sauce in a resealable plastic bag. Place the bag in the refrigerator and let the fish marinate for 30 minutes.
2. Once marinated, bring the water to a boil in a large pot over high heat. Add the cabbage and onion and bring to a boil again.
3. Add the tofu, marinated fish, and any remaining marinade to the pot.
4. Bring the soup back to a boil, reduce the heat to medium, and simmer for 5 minutes, until fragrant. Serve immediately.

Nutrition Info:

- Per Serving: Calories :181 ; Fat: 4g ;Saturated fat: 1g ;Sodium: 271 mg

Fresh Creamy Fruit Dip

Servings: 6

Cooking Time: X

Ingredients:

- 1 (3-ounce) package light cream cheese, softened
- 1 cup vanilla yogurt
- 2 tablespoons honey
- 2 tablespoons orange juice
- 2 tablespoons brown sugar

Directions:

1. In medium bowl, beat cream cheese until light and fluffy. Gradually add yogurt, beating until smooth. Add honey, orange juice, and brown sugar and beat well. Cover and chill for at least 4 hours before serving.

Nutrition Info:

- Per Serving: Calories: 99.31; Fat:3.14g ;Saturated fat:1.98 g ;Sodium: 72.66 mg

Spicy Lentil Chili

Servings: 4

Cooking Time: 20 Minutes

Ingredients:

- 1 tablespoon olive oil
- 1 onion, chopped
- 5 cloves garlic, minced
- 1 jalapeño pepper, seeded and minced
- 1 cup red lentils, sorted and rinsed
- 1 tablespoon chili powder
- 1 teaspoon smoked paprika
- 1/8 teaspoon red pepper flakes
- 1 (14-ounce) can no-salt-added diced tomatoes, undrained
- 3 tablespoons no-salt-added tomato paste
- 1 (16-ounce) can low-sodium kidney beans, rinsed and drained
- 1/3 cup chopped fresh cilantro leaves

Directions:

1. In a large saucepan, heat the olive oil over medium heat.
2. Add the onion, garlic, and jalapeño pepper, and cook and stir for 2 minutes.
3. Add the lentils, chili powder, paprika, red pepper flakes, tomatoes, tomato paste, and kidney beans, and bring to a boil.
4. Lower the heat, partially cover the pan, and simmer for 15 to 18 minutes, or until the chili powder has blended in and the lentils are tender. Top with the fresh cilantro and serve.

Nutrition Info:

- Per Serving: Calories: 364; Fat: 5g ;Saturated fat: 1g ;Sodium:130 mg

Broccoli And Carrot Salad With Dried Cranberries

Servings: X

Cooking Time: X

Ingredients:

- For the dressing
- 3 tablespoons apple cider vinegar
- 2 tablespoons olive oil
- 1 tablespoon honey
- 1 teaspoon chopped fresh thyme
- Sea salt
- Freshly ground black pepper
- For the salad
- 2 cups broccoli slaw
- 2 carrots, shredded
- 1 red bell pepper, julienned
- 1 yellow bell pepper, julienned
- 2 cups shredded kale
- 2 tablespoons dried cranberries
- 2 tablespoons sliced or slivered almonds

Directions:

1. To make the dressing
2. In a small bowl, whisk together the vinegar, olive oil, honey, and thyme until well blended.
3. Season with salt and pepper and set aside
4. To make the salad
5. In a medium bowl, mix together the broccoli, carrots, bell peppers, kale, cranberries, and almonds and toss with the dressing until combined.
6. Serve.

Nutrition Info:

- Per Serving: Calories: 358; Fat: 18g ;Saturated fat: 2 g ;Sodium: 84 mg

German Potato Soup

Servings: 4

Cooking Time: 20 Minutes

Ingredients:

- 2 teaspoons olive oil
- 2 onions, chopped
- 4 cloves garlic, minced
- 2 large Yukon Gold potatoes, rinsed and chopped
- 2 cups low-sodium vegetable broth
- 1 tablespoon low-sodium yellow mustard
- 1 teaspoon tamari sauce
- 1 tablespoon chopped fresh rosemary leaves
- ½ teaspoon dried sage leaves
- ¼ cup plain low-fat Greek yogurt
- ¼ cup grated extra sharp cheddar cheese
- ⅓ cup chopped fresh flat-leaf parsley
- ¼ cup vegan bacon bits (optional)

Directions:

1. In a large saucepan, heat the olive oil over medium heat.
2. Add the onions and garlic, and cook and stir for 3 minutes.
3. Add the potatoes, vegetable broth, mustard, tamari, rosemary, and sage, and bring to a simmer. Simmer for 14 to 17 minutes or until the potatoes are tender.
4. At this point, some of the soup needs to be puréed, and there are many methods you can choose from. You can do this with an immersion blender, leaving some of the potato chunks whole if you'd like. You can use a potato masher right in the pot. Or put half of the soup into a blender, cover the blender with the lid and a towel, and blend until smooth. Then pour the blended mixture back into the soup. After you have puréed the soup, stir in the yogurt and cheddar cheese.
5. Simmer the soup for 1 minute, then ladle into bowls. Garnish with the parsley and vegan bacon bits, if using.

Nutrition Info:

- Per Serving: Calories:223; Fat: 5g ;Saturated fat: 2g ;Sodium:208 mg

Spicy Butter Beans

Servings: 2

Cooking Time: 15 Min

Ingredients:

- 1 tsp olive oil
- ½ cup red onion, chopped
- ½ jalapeño pepper, chopped
- 1 tsp garlic, crushed
- 1 (16 oz) can butter beans, rinsed and drained
- ¼ tsp ground cumin
- ⅛ tsp ground coriander
- ¼ tsp red pepper flakes (optional)
- 1 tsp parsley, chopped for garnish
- Himalayan pink salt
- Ground black pepper

Directions:

1. Warm the olive oil in a medium-sized stockpot over medium-high heat.
2. Add the garlic, ginger, cumin, and coriander and fry for 2 minutes until fragrant.
3. Mix in the carrots, vegetable broth, lemon juice, and honey. Boil the mixture, reduce the heat to low, and simmer for 6 to 8 minutes until the carrots are tender.
4. Season with salt and pepper, serve immediately.

Nutrition Info:

- Per Serving: Calories: 291 ; Fat:1 g ;Saturated fat: 0g ;Sodium: 34 mg

Corn Polenta Chowder

Servings: 6

Cooking Time: X

Ingredients:

- 2 strips turkey bacon
- 1 tablespoon olive oil
- 1 red onion, chopped
- 3 cloves garlic, minced
- 1 red bell pepper, chopped
- 2 jalapeño peppers, minced
- 2 Yukon Gold potatoes, chopped
- 5 cups Low-Sodium Chicken Broth , divided
- 1/3 cup cornmeal
- 2 tablespoons adobo sauce
- 2 (10-ounce) packages frozen corn, thawed
- 1 cup fat-free half-and-half
- ¼ cup chopped cilantro
- 1/8 teaspoon cayenne pepper

Directions:

1. In large soup pot, cook bacon until crisp. Remove from heat, crumble, and set aside. To drippings remaining in pot, add olive oil, then onion and garlic; cook and stir until tender, about 5 minutes.
2. Stir in bell peppers, jalapeños, potatoes, and 3 cups of the broth. Bring to a boil, then reduce heat, cover, and simmer for 20 minutes until potatoes are tender.
3. Meanwhile, in small microwave-safe bowl, combine cornmeal and 1 cup chicken broth. Microwave on high for 2 minutes, remove and stir, then microwave for 2–4 minutes longer or until mixture thickens; stir in adobo sauce and remaining 1 cup chicken broth. Add to soup along with corn. Simmer for another 10 minutes.
4. Add the half-and-half, cilantro, and pepper and stir well. Heat until steam rises, then sprinkle with reserved bacon and serve immediately.

Nutrition Info:

- Per Serving: Calories: 276.10 ; Fat: 6.03 g ;Saturated fat:1.42g ;Sodium: 184.32 mg

Greek Quesadillas

Servings: 8

Cooking Time: X

Ingredients:

- 1 cucumber
- 1 cup plain yogurt
- ½ teaspoon dried oregano leaves
- 1 tablespoon lemon juice
- ½ cup crumbled feta cheese
- 4 green onions, chopped
- 3 plum tomatoes, chopped
- 1 cup fresh baby spinach leaves
- 1 cup shredded part-skim mozzarella cheese
- 12 (6-inch) no-salt corn tortillas

Directions:

1. Peel cucumber, remove seeds, and chop. In small bowl, combine cucumber with yogurt, oregano, and lemon juice and set aside.
2. In medium bowl, combine feta cheese, green onions, tomatoes, baby spinach, and mozzarella cheese and mix well.
3. Preheat griddle or skillet. Place six tortillas on work surface. Divide tomato mixture among them. Top with remaining tortillas and press down gently.
4. Cook quesadillas, pressing down occasionally with spatula, until tortillas are lightly browned. Flip quesadillas and cook on second side until tortillas are crisp and cheese is melted. Cut quesadillas in quarters and serve with yogurt mixture.

Nutrition Info:

- Per Serving: Calories:181.26 ; Fat: 6.34 g ;Saturated fat:3.62 g ;Sodium: 208.14 mg

Spring Asparagus Soup

Servings: 4

Cooking Time: X

Ingredients:

- 1 tablespoon olive oil
- 3 scallions, chopped
- ½ cup finely chopped sweet onion
- 1 clove garlic, minced
- 2 new potatoes, peeled and chopped
- 1 pound asparagus
- 4 cups Low-Sodium Chicken Broth
- 1 tablespoon lemon juice
- 1 teaspoon lemon zest
- 1 tablespoon fresh thyme leaves
- 1/8 teaspoon white pepper
- 1 cup fat-free half-and-half

Directions:

1. In large soup pot, heat olive oil over medium heat. Add scallions, sweet onion, and garlic; cook and stir for 3 minutes. Then add potatoes; cook and stir for 5 minutes longer.
2. Snap the asparagus spears and discard ends. Chop asparagus into 1″ pieces and add to pot along with broth. Bring to a boil, reduce heat, cover, and simmer for 10 minutes.
3. Using an immersion blender, puree the soup until smooth. Add lemon juice, lemon zest, thyme, pepper, and half-and-half, heat until steaming, and serve. You can also serve this soup chilled. (Without an immersion blender, puree the soup in four batches in a blender or food processor, then return to the pot and continue with the recipe.)

Nutrition Info:

- Per Serving: Calories:201.50 ; Fat: 6.04 g ;Saturated fat:1.52 g ;Sodium: 182.69 mg

Garbanzo Bean Salad

Servings: 6

Cooking Time: 15 Min

Ingredients:

- 3 tbsp. avocado olive oil, divided
- 2 tbsp. balsamic vinegar
- ½ tsp fine sea salt, divided
- ¼ tsp ground black pepper
- 1 cup Israeli couscous
- 1 cup water
- 2 cups grape tomatoes, halved
- ¼ cup black olives, pitted and sliced
- 1 (15 oz) can garbanzo beans, drained and rinsed
- ¼ cup parsley, chopped

Directions:

1. In a small Pyrex jug, add 2 tbsp. of avocado oil, balsamic vinegar, ¼ tsp salt, and black pepper, whisk to combine. Set aside.
2. Heat the remaining 1 tbsp. avocado oil in a large heavy-bottom pan over medium-high heat.
3. Add the Israeli couscous and cook for 2 minutes, stirring frequently, until lightly browned. Add the water and allow to boil.
4. Mix in the remaining ¼ tsp salt. Reduce the heat to low and simmer. Cook for 10 minutes, or until tender. Remove from the heat and drain. Set aside to cool.
5. In a large-sized serving bowl, add the tomato halves, garbanzo beans, and the vinaigrette, mix to combine.
6. Add the cooked couscous and mix to incorporate. Leave it to cool to room temperature.
7. Mix in the chopped parsley and serve.

Nutrition Info:

- Per Serving: Calories: 231 ; Fat:8g ;Saturated fat: 1g ;Sodium: 282 mg

butternut Squash And Lentil Soup

Servings: 4

Cooking Time: 20 Minutes

Ingredients:

- 1 tablespoon olive oil
- 1 onion, chopped
- 1 tablespoon peeled grated fresh ginger root
- 1 (12-ounce) package peeled and diced butternut squash
- 1 cup red lentils, rinsed and sorted
- 5 cups low-sodium vegetable broth
- 1 cup unsweetened apple juice
- Pinch salt
- ⅛ teaspoon black pepper
- ¼ teaspoon curry powder
- 1 sprig fresh thyme
- 3 tablespoons crumbled blue cheese

Directions:

1. In a large saucepan, heat the olive oil over medium heat. Add the onion, and cook and stir for 3 minutes. Add the ginger, squash, and lentils, and cook and stir for 1 minute.
2. Turn up the heat to medium-high, and add the broth, apple juice, salt, pepper, curry powder, and thyme. Bring the mixture to a boil.
3. Reduce the heat to low and partially cover the pan. Simmer for 15 to 18 minutes or until the squash and lentils are tender. Remove the thyme sprig; the leaves will have fallen off.
4. Purée the soup, either in a food processor, with an immersion blender, or with a potato masher. Heat again, then ladle into bowls, sprinkle with the blue cheese, and serve warm.

Nutrition Info:

- Per Serving: Calories: 317 ; Fat: 7g ;Saturated fat: 2g ;Sodium:280 mg

Fresh Yellow-tomato Soup

Servings: 6

Cooking Time: X

Ingredients:

- 8 yellow tomatoes
- 1 tablespoon olive oil
- 1 tablespoon butter
- 4 cloves garlic, peeled and minced
- 1 yellow bell pepper, chopped
- 1 red bell pepper, chopped
- 4 cups Low-Sodium Chicken Broth
- 1 tablespoon lemon juice
- 1/8 teaspoon white pepper
- 1 large bunch basil, torn
- ¼ cup toasted sliced almonds

Directions:

1. Prepare large bowl of ice water. Bring large pot of water to a boil. Cut X into bottom of each tomato and drop tomatoes into boiling water. Bring water back to a boil and simmer for 1 minute, then remove each tomato and drop into ice water. Let cool for 5 minutes, then peel tomatoes; discard skin.
2. Heat large soup pot over medium heat and add olive oil and butter and let melt. Add garlic; cook and stir for 3 minutes. Cut tomatoes into quarters and add to pot along with peppers. Cook and stir for 4 minutes.
3. Add the broth, lemon juice, and pepper. Bring to a boil and cook for 10 minutes, then add half of the basil.
4. Using an immersion blender, puree soup. Or puree soup in batches in a blender or food processor. Garnish with remaining basil and toasted almonds and serve.

Nutrition Info:

- Per Serving: Calories:197.11 ; Fat: 11.57 g ;Saturated fat: 3.08 g;Sodium: 158.84 mg

Buttermilk Dressing

Servings: 4

Cooking Time: X

Ingredients:

- ¼ cup buttermilk
- 2 tablespoons low-fat mayonnaise
- 2 tablespoons lemon juice
- 2 shallots, chopped
- ¼ teaspoon salt
- 1 tablespoon chopped chives
- 1 tablespoon chopped fresh dill
- 1/8 teaspoon pepper

Directions:

1. Combine all ingredients in blender or food processor and blend or process until mixed. Cover and store in refrigerator for up to 4 days.

Nutrition Info:

- Per Serving: Calories:28.37; Fat:1.46 g ;Saturated fat: 0.31 g;Sodium: 124.09 mg

Sweet Garlic-vinegar Crushed Cucumber

Servings: 2

Cooking Time: 15 Minutes

Ingredients:

- 1 English cucumber
- 1 tablespoon minced garlic
- 1 tablespoon vinegar
- 1 teaspoon sugar
- 1 teaspoon sesame oil
- Pinch sea salt

Directions:

1. Place the cucumber in plastic wrap or a resealable plastic bag, put it on a flat surface, and lightly smash it with a hard object, such as a skillet, rolling pin, or mallet.
2. Remove the plastic wrap and slice the crushed cucumber into 1-inch slices.
3. In a medium bowl, mix the cucumber with the garlic, vinegar, sugar, sesame oil, and a pinch of salt. Enjoy immediately.

Nutrition Info:

- Per Serving: Calories: 58 ; Fat: 2 g ;Saturated fat: 0 g ;Sodium: 81 mg

Honey-garlic Chicken Stew

Servings: 5

Cooking Time: 25 Minutes

Ingredients:

- 1 tablespoon olive oil
- 1 pound boneless, skinless chicken thighs, cut into bite-size pieces
- ⅓ cup Honey-Garlic Sauce
- 1 tablespoon white vinegar
- 1 cup chopped carrots
- 1 white onion, chopped
- 1 cup water

Directions:

1. In a large skillet, heat the olive oil over high heat and add the chicken, Honey-Garlic Sauce, and vinegar and cook for about 5 minutes, or until the chicken is cooked through and no longer pink.
2. Add the carrots and onion and sauté until the onion is translucent, about 2 minutes.
3. Add the water and bring the stew to a boil, reduce the heat to medium, and simmer for 15 minutes until the water mostly evaporates. Serve immediately.

Nutrition Info:

- Per Serving: Calories: 195 ; Fat: 9g ;Saturated fat: 1g ;Sodium: 310 mg

Garbanzo Bean Pops

Servings: 4

Cooking Time: 30 Min

Ingredients:

- Aluminum foil
- 1 (15 oz) can garbanzo beans, drained and rinsed
- 1 tsp avocado oil
- ¼ tsp ground cumin
- ¼ tsp paprika
- Pinch red pepper flakes
- Himalayan pink Salt
- Ground black pepper

Directions:

1. Heat the oven to 400°F gas mark 6. Line a baking sheet with aluminum foil.
2. Use a clean tea towel to dry the garbanzo beans well. Discard any loose skin.
3. Place the garbanzo beans on the baking sheet and drizzle with avocado oil, toss to coat.
4. Place the baking sheet in the oven and roast for 25 to 30 minutes, until the garbanzo beans are crispy and browned. Remove from the oven.
5. Add the cumin, paprika, red pepper flakes, salt and pepper to taste, toss to combine.

Nutrition Info:

- Per Serving: Calories: 89 ; Fat:3 g ;Saturated fat: 0g ;Sodium: 160 mg

Low-sodium Chicken Broth

Servings: 8

Cooking Time: X

Ingredients:

- 2 tablespoons olive oil
- 3 pounds cut-up chicken
- 2 onions, chopped
- 5 cloves garlic, minced
- 4 carrots, sliced
- 4 stalks celery, sliced
- 1 tablespoon peppercorns
- 1 bay leaf
- 6 cups water
- 2 tablespoons lemon juice

Directions:

1. In large skillet, heat olive oil over medium heat. Add chicken, skin-side down, and cook until browned, about 8–10 minutes. Place chicken in 5- to 6-quart slow cooker.
2. Add onions and garlic to drippings in skillet; cook and stir for 2–3 minutes, scraping bottom of skillet. Add to slow cooker along with remaining ingredients except lemon juice. Cover and cook on low for 8–9 hours.
3. Strain broth into large bowl. Remove meat from chicken; refrigerate or freeze for another use. Cover broth and refrigerate overnight. In the morning, remove fat solidified on surface and discard. Stir in lemon juice. Pour broth into freezer containers, seal, label, and freeze up to 3 months. To use, defrost in refrigerator overnight.

Nutrition Info:

- Per Serving: Calories: 82.89 ; Fat: 5.22g ;Saturated fat:0.92 mg;Sodium: 39.09 mg

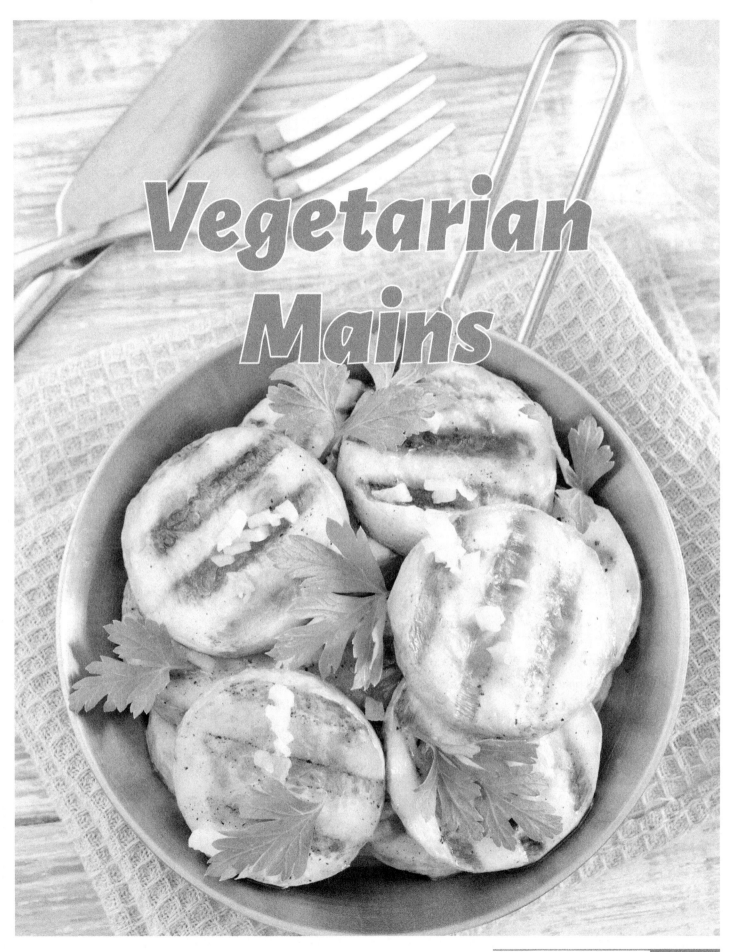

Vegetarian Mains

Vegetarian Mains

Broccoli Stuffed Sweetato

Servings: 4

Cooking Time: 30 Min

Ingredients:

- 4 large sweet potatoes, washed
- 1 tbsp. avocado oil, divided
- 2 cups broccoli florets
- Himalayan pink salt
- Ground black pepper
- 1 (15 oz) can low-sodium black-eyed peas, drained and rinsed
- ½ cup organic tahini dressing
- 2 spring onions, finely sliced

Directions:

1. Heat the oven to 375°F gas mark 5.
2. Use a fork to pierce the sweet potatoes all over.
3. Rub the sweet potato skin with ½ tbsp. of avocado oil and place them on a baking sheet.
4. Bake for 20 to 30 minutes, or until fully cooked and easily pierced with a fork.
5. In a medium-sized mixing bowl, add the broccoli and the remaining ½ tbsp. of avocado oil, toss to coat. Season with salt and pepper to taste.
6. After 10 minutes of baking the sweet potatoes, arrange the seasoned broccoli onto the baking sheet and roast for 20 minutes, or until tender and lightly browned. Remove from the oven.
7. Cut the sweet potatoes in half lengthwise, top with the black-eyed peas and roasted broccoli.
8. Drizzle with the tahini dressing and sprinkle spring onion on top. Serve warm.

Nutrition Info:

- Per Serving: Calories: 368 ; Fat: 15 g ;Saturated fat: 2 g ;Sodium: 564 mg

Curried Garbanzo Beans

Servings: 4

Cooking Time: 15 Min

Ingredients:

- 2 tbsp. coconut oil
- 1 tbsp. garlic, crushed
- 1 (15 oz) can low-sodium garbanzo beans, drained and rinsed
- 1 (15 oz) can low-sodium diced tomatoes with their juices
- 1 tsp mild or hot curry powder
- ½ tsp fine sea salt
- ¼ tsp ground black pepper
- 4 cups baby spinach

Directions:

1. In a large, heavy-bottom pan, heat the coconut oil over medium heat.
2. Add the garlic and cook for 20 seconds, until fragrant.
3. Add the garbanzo beans, tomatoes with their juices, mild or hot curry powder, fine sea salt and pepper, mix to combine. Simmer for 10 minutes, stirring regularly, or until the flavours come together.
4. Add the baby spinach and stir for 1 to 2 minutes, until the spinach has wilted. Remove from the heat and serve immediately.

Nutrition Info:

- Per Serving: Calories: 168 ; Fat: 9 g ;Saturated fat: 1 g ;Sodium: 352 mg

Tofu And Root Vegetable Curry

Servings: X

Cooking Time: 25 Minutes

Ingredients:

- 2 teaspoons olive oil
- 1 cup small cauliflower florets
- 1 parsnip, diced
- 1 carrot, diced
- 1 red bell pepper, thinly sliced
- 1 cup diced sweet potato
- 1 teaspoon peeled, grated fresh ginger
- ½ teaspoon minced garlic
- 1 cup low-sodium vegetable broth
- 2 tomatoes, chopped
- 2 cups diced extra-firm tofu
- 2 tablespoons curry powder or paste
- ¼ cup chopped cashews, for garnish

Directions:

1. In a large saucepan, warm the olive oil over medium-high heat.
2. Add the cauliflower, parsnips, carrots, bell peppers, sweet potatoes, ginger, and garlic and sauté until the vegetables begin to soften, about 10 minutes.
3. Stir in the vegetable broth, tomatoes, tofu, and curry powder and bring the mixture to a boil.
4. Reduce the heat to low and simmer until the vegetables are tender and everything is completely heated through, 15 to 18 minutes.
5. Serve topped with cashews.

Nutrition Info:

- Per Serving: Calories: 457 ; Fat: 20 g ;Saturated fat: 3 g ;Sodium: 135 mg

Butternut Squash, Bulgur, And Tempeh Burritos

Servings: X

Cooking Time: 15 Minutes

Ingredients:

- 1 teaspoon olive oil
- 1 cup chopped butternut squash
- ½ cup chopped onion
- ½ cup cooked bulgur
- ½ cup crumbled tempeh
- ½ teaspoon chili powder
- ¼ teaspoon ground cumin
- 4 (6-inch) whole-grain tortillas
- ½ cup low-sodium tomato or mango salsa
- 1 scallion, white and green parts, sliced
- ½ cup shredded lettuce
- ¼ cup fat-free sour cream

Directions:

1. In a medium skillet, warm the olive oil over medium-high heat.
2. Add the squash and onions and sauté until tender, 8 to 10 minutes.
3. Add the bulgur, tempeh, chili powder, and cumin and sauté until the bulgur is heated through, about 7 minutes.
4. Wrap the tortillas in a clean kitchen towel and heat in the microwave for 15 to 30 seconds.
5. Lay the tortillas out and evenly divide the squash mixture between them. Top each with the salsa, scallion, lettuce, and sour cream.
6. Wrap the tortillas around the filling and serve.

Nutrition Info:

- Per Serving: Calories: 423 ; Fat: 13 g ;Saturated fat: 2 g ;Sodium: 712 mg

Corn-and-chili Pancakes

Servings: 6

Cooking Time: X

Ingredients:

- ½ cup buttermilk
- 1 tablespoon olive oil
- ½ cup egg substitute
- ½ cup grated extra-sharp Cheddar cheese
- 1 jalapeño pepper, minced
- 2 ears sweet corn
- ½ cup cornmeal
- 1 cup all-purpose flour
- 1½ teaspoons baking powder
- ½ teaspoon baking soda
- 1 tablespoon sugar
- 1 tablespoon chili powder
- 1 tablespoon peanut oil
- 1 tablespoon butter

Directions:

1. In large bowl, combine buttermilk, olive oil, egg substitute, Cheddar, and jalapeño pepper and mix well.
2. Cut the kernels off the sweet corn and add to buttermilk mixture along with cornmeal, flour, baking powder, baking soda, sugar, and chili powder; mix until combined. Let stand for 10 minutes.
3. Heat griddle or frying pan over medium heat. Brush with the butter, then add the batter, ¼ cup at a time. Cook until bubbles form and start to break and sides look dry, about 3–4 minutes. Carefully flip pancakes and cook until light golden brown on second side, about 2–3 minutes. Serve immediately.

Nutrition Info:

- Per Serving: Calories:252.62; Fat: 9.20 g ;Saturated fat:3.03 g ;Sodium:287.01 mg

Portobello Burgers

Servings: 4

Cooking Time: 25 Min

Ingredients:

- Aluminium foil
- 3 tbsp. avocado oil
- 1 tbsp. garlic, crushed
- 4 large portobello mushrooms, stems removed
- 4 crusty whole-grain rolls
- ½ cup dairy-free cheddar cheese, shredded
- Ground black pepper
- 4 iceberg lettuce leaves

Directions:

1. Heat the oven to 425°F gas mark 7. Line a baking sheet with aluminum foil.
2. In a small-sized mixing bowl, add the avocado oil and garlic, mix to combine. Brush half of the garlic mixture on both sides of the portobello mushrooms and let them sit for 10 minutes.
3. Meanwhile, cut the rolls open. Drizzle the remaining garlic mixture onto the bottom half of each roll. Place 2 tbsp. of cheddar cheese on each bottom half roll.
4. Place the mushrooms on the prepared baking sheet, cap-side down, and roast for 12 minutes on each side.
5. Put one portobello mushroom on the bottom of each roll, on top of the cheddar cheese. Season with ground black pepper and top with 1 lettuce leaf. Place the top bun on the lettuce leaf and serve. Repeat for the remaining mushrooms.

Nutrition Info:

- Per Serving: Calories: 307 ; Fat: 17 g ;Saturated fat: 5 g ;Sodium: 276 mg

Pumpkin And Chickpea Patties

Servings: X

Cooking Time: 20 Minutes

Ingredients:

- 2 teaspoons olive oil, divided
- 2 cups grated fresh pumpkin
- ½ cup grated carrot
- ½ teaspoon minced garlic
- 2 cups low-sodium chickpeas, rinsed and drained
- ½ cup ground almonds
- 2 large egg whites
- 1 scallion, white and green parts, chopped
- ½ teaspoon chopped fresh thyme
- Sea salt
- Freshly ground black pepper

Directions:

1. Preheat the oven to 400°F.
2. Line a baking sheet with parchment paper and set aside.
3. In a large skillet, heat ½ teaspoon olive oil over medium-high heat. Add the pumpkin, carrots, and garlic and sauté until softened, about 4 minutes. Remove from the heat and transfer to a food processor. Wipe the skillet clean with paper towels.
4. Add the chickpeas, almonds, egg whites, scallions, and thyme to the food processor. Pulse until the mixture holds together when pressed.
5. Season with salt and pepper and divide the pumpkin mixture into 8 equal patties, flattening them to about ½-inch thick.
6. Heat the remaining 1½ teaspoons olive oil in the skillet. Cook the patties until lightly browned, about 4 minutes on each side.
7. Place the skillet in the oven and bake for an additional 5 minutes, until the patties are completely heated through.
8. Serve.

Nutrition Info:

- Per Serving: Calories: 560 ; Fat: 25 g ;Saturated fat: 3 g ;Sodium: 62 mg

Risotto With Artichokes

Servings: 6

Cooking Time: X

Ingredients:

- 2 cups water
- 2½ cups low-sodium vegetable broth
- 2 tablespoons olive oil
- 4 shallots, minced
- 3 cloves garlic, minced
- 1 (10-ounce) box frozen artichoke hearts, thawed
- 1½ cups Arborio rice
- 1/8 teaspoon pepper
- ¼ cup grated Parmesan cheese
- 1 tablespoon butter
- ½ cup chopped fresh basil leaves

Directions:

1. In medium saucepan, combine water and broth; heat over low heat until warm; keep on heat.
2. In large saucepan, heat olive oil over medium heat. Add shallots and garlic; cook and stir until crisp-tender, about 4 minutes. Add artichokes; cook and stir for 3 minutes.
3. Add rice; cook and stir for 2 minutes. Add the broth mixture, a cup at a time, stirring until the liquid is absorbed, about 20–25 minutes. Stir in pepper, Parmesan, butter, and basil; cover and let stand for 5 minutes off the heat. Serve immediately.

Nutrition Info:

- Per Serving: Calories:317.17 ; Fat: 8.90 g ;Saturated fat:2.86g ;Sodium: 223.71 mg

Cauliflower, Green Pea, And Wild Rice Pilaf

Servings: X

Cooking Time: 45 Minutes

Ingredients:

- 2 teaspoons olive oil
- ½ small sweet onion, chopped
- 1 teaspoon minced garlic
- 1 cup wild rice
- 3½ cups low-sodium vegetable broth
- 1 cup small cauliflower florets
- 1 cup frozen green peas
- ½ cup low-sodium canned lentils, rinsed and drained
- 1 teaspoon chopped fresh thyme
- 2 tablespoons sunflower seeds

Directions:

1. In a large skillet, warm the olive oil over medium-high heat.
2. Add the onions and garlic and sauté until softened, about 3 minutes.
3. Stir in the rice and broth and bring to a boil. Reduce the heat to low, cover, and let simmer until most of the liquid is absorbed and the rice is tender, about 45 minutes.
4. While the rice is cooking, place a medium saucepan filled with water over high heat and bring to a boil. Add the cauliflower and peas and blanch until tender-crisp, about 5 minutes. Drain and set aside.
5. When the rice is cooked, stir in the lentils, cauliflower, peas, thyme, and sunflower seeds.
6. Serve.

Nutrition Info:

- Per Serving: Calories: 565 ; Fat: 9 g ;Saturated fat: 1 g ;Sodium: 150 mg

Spinach-ricotta Omelet

Servings: 4

Cooking Time: X

Ingredients:

- 1 (10-ounce) package frozen chopped spinach, thawed and drained
- ½ cup part-skim ricotta cheese
- 2 tablespoons grated Parmesan cheese
- 1/8 teaspoon nutmeg
- 7 egg whites
- 1 egg yolk
- ¼ cup milk
- 1/8 teaspoon pepper
- 1 tablespoon olive oil
- ¼ cup finely chopped onion

Directions:

1. Press spinach between layers of paper towel to remove all excess moisture. Set aside. In small bowl, combine ricotta with Parmesan cheese and nutmeg; set aside.
2. In medium bowl, beat egg whites until a soft foam forms. In small bowl, combine egg yolk with milk and pepper and beat well.
3. Heat a nonstick skillet over medium heat. Add olive oil, then add spinach and onion; cook and stir until onion is crisp-tender, about 4 minutes. Meanwhile, fold egg-yolk mixture into beaten egg whites. Add egg mixture to skillet; cook, running spatula around edges to let uncooked mixture flow underneath, until eggs are set but still moist.
4. Spoon ricotta mixture on top of eggs; cover pan, and let cook for 2 minutes. Then fold omelet and serve immediately.

Nutrition Info:

- Per Serving: Calories: 162.81; Fat:8.74 g ;Saturated fat: 3.23 g ;Sodium: 245.82 mg

Stuffed Noodle Squash

Servings: 4

Cooking Time: 50 Min

Ingredients:

- 2 small spaghetti squash, halved lengthwise and seeds removed
- 1 cup water
- Aluminum foil
- 2 tbsp. olive oil
- 2 cups spinach, stems removed and finely chopped
- 1 cup chayote squash, peeled and chopped
- 1 cup canned garbanzo bean, drained and rinsed
- ¼ tsp fine sea salt
- ¼ tsp ground black pepper
- 1 cup Marinara Sauce

Directions:

1. Heat the oven to 400°F gas mark 6.
2. Place the spaghetti squashes cut side down on a large baking sheet.
3. Add the water to the baking sheet and cover it with aluminum foil. Bake for 35 to 40 minutes, or until the squash is fully cooked. Remove from the oven, leaving the oven on.
4. In a large, heavy-bottom pan, heat the olive oil over a medium heat.
5. Add the spinach and fry for 2 to 3 minutes until wilted.
6. Add the chayote squash and garbanzo beans, cook for 2 minutes until heated through.
7. Use a fork to scrape the flesh from the squash to remove the strands. Keep the shells.
8. Mix the strands into the garbanzo beans mixture and season with salt and pepper. Divide the mixture into the squash shells.
9. Drizzle each shell with ¼ cup Marinara Sauce. Return the stuffed squash to the oven and bake for 10 minutes until heated through. Serve hot.

Nutrition Info:

- Per Serving: Calories: 252 ; Fat: 13 g ;Saturated fat: 2 g ;Sodium: 330 mg

Stuffed Mushrooms

Servings: 4

Cooking Time: 10 Min

Ingredients:

- 4 large portobello mushrooms, stems removed
- 1 tbsp. avocado oil
- 1 (15 oz) can low-sodium garbanzo beans, drained and rinsed
- 1 cup wild rice, cooked
- ½ medium red bell pepper, seeds removed and finely chopped
- ½ cup red cabbage, finely chopped
- Himalayan pink salt
- Ground black pepper

Directions:

1. Heat the oven to 350°F gas mark 4.
2. Place the portobello mushrooms gill side down on a large baking sheet and drizzle with avocado oil.
3. Bake for 10 minutes, flip, and bake for another 10 minutes, until tender. Remove and leave the oven on.
4. In a large-sized mixing bowl, add the garbanzo beans, wild rice, red bell pepper, and red cabbage, season with salt and pepper to taste.
5. Divide the mixture into each portobello mushroom cup. Return to the oven and bake for 10 minutes until heated through. Remove from the oven and serve warm.

Nutrition Info:

- Per Serving: Calories: 194 ; Fat: 6 g ;Saturated fat: 1 g ;Sodium: 181 mg

Spaghetti Squash Skillet

Servings: X

Cooking Time: 35 Minutes

Ingredients:

- 1 (2-pound) spaghetti squash
- 1 tablespoon olive oil, divided
- Sea salt
- Freshly ground black pepper
- ½ cup chopped sweet onion
- 1 teaspoon minced garlic
- 1 orange bell pepper, diced
- 16 asparagus spears, woody ends trimmed, cut into 2-inch pieces
- ½ cup sliced sun-dried tomatoes
- 2 cups shredded kale
- 1 tablespoon chopped fresh basil

Directions:

1. Preheat the oven to 400°F.
2. Line a baking sheet with parchment paper and set aside.
3. Slice the squash in half lengthwise and scoop out the seeds. Place the squash, cut-side up, on the baking sheet. Brush the cut edges and hollows with 1 teaspoon olive oil and season lightly with salt and pepper.
4. Roast the squash until a knife can be inserted easily into the thickest section, 30 to 35 minutes.
5. Remove from the oven and let the squash cool for 10 minutes, then use a fork to shred the flesh into a medium bowl. Set aside.
6. While the squash is cooling, warm the remaining 2 teaspoons olive oil in a medium skillet over medium heat. Add the onions and garlic and sauté until softened, about 3 minutes.
7. Stir in the bell pepper, asparagus, sun-dried tomatoes, and kale and sauté until the vegetables and greens are tender, about 5 minutes.
8. Add the shredded spaghetti squash and basil and toss to combine.
9. Serve.

Nutrition Info:

- Per Serving: Calories: 340 ; Fat:10 g ;Saturated fat: 2 g ;Sodium: 287 mg

Garbanzo Sandwich

Servings: 4

Cooking Time: 10 Min

Ingredients:

- 1 (15 oz) can low-sodium garbanzo bean, drained and rinsed
- ¼ cup medium red onion, finely chopped
- ¼ cup plain unsweetened coconut milk yoghurt
- 1½ tsp whole-grain mustard
- Himalayan pink salt
- Ground black pepper
- 2 green leaf lettuce leaves
- 4 whole-grain bread slices

Directions:

1. In a medium-sized mixing bowl, use a fork to mash up the garbanzo beans roughly. There must be some chunky pieces.
2. Add the red onion, coconut milk yoghurt, and wholegrain mustard. Season with salt and pepper to taste, mix to combine.
3. Place 1 green leaf lettuce leaf on each of the 2 wholegrain bread slices. Divide the garbanzo bean mixture between the 2 slices of bread on top of the lettuce leaf.
4. Top with the remaining slice of bread and serve.

Nutrition Info:

- Per Serving: Calories: 162; Fat: 3 g ;Saturated fat: 1 g ;Sodium: 287mg

Rice-and-vegetable Casserole

Servings: 8

Cooking Time: X

Ingredients:

- 1 tablespoon olive oil
- 2 onions, chopped
- 1 (8-ounce) package sliced mushrooms
- 2 red bell peppers, chopped
- 1 jalapeño pepper, minced
- 4 cups cooked brown rice
- 1½ cups milk
- 1 egg
- 2 egg whites
- ½ cup low-fat sour cream
- 1 cup shredded part-skim mozzarella cheese
- ½ cup shredded Colby cheese

Directions:

1. Preheat oven to 350ºF. Spray a 13″ × 9″ baking pan with nonstick cooking spray and set aside.
2. In large saucepan, heat olive oil. Add onions and mushrooms; cook and stir for 3 minutes. Then add bell peppers and jalapeño pepper; cook and stir for 3–4 minutes longer until vegetables are crisp-tender.
3. In large bowl, combine rice, milk, egg, egg whites, sour cream, mozzarella cheese, and Colby cheese. Layer half of this mixture in the prepared baking pan. Top with vegetables, then top with remaining rice mixture. Bake for 50–65 minutes or until casserole is bubbling, set, and beginning to brown. Let stand for 5 minutes, then cut into squares to serve.

Nutrition Info:

- Per Serving: Calories:276.42; Fat:10.87 g ;Saturated fat:5.35 g ;Sodium: 175.20 mg

Smoky Bean And Lentil Chili

Servings: X

Cooking Time: 30 Minutes

Ingredients:

- 1 teaspoon olive oil
- 1 red bell pepper, diced
- ¼ cup chopped sweet onion
- 1 teaspoon minced garlic
- 2 tablespoons chili powder
- 1 teaspoon smoked sweet paprika
- 1 cup low-sodium canned black beans, rinsed and drained
- 1 cup low-sodium canned lentils, rinsed and drained
- 1 cup shelled edamame
- 1 cup low-sodium canned diced tomatoes, drained
- ½ cup corn kernels
- ½ diced avocado, for garnish

Directions:

1. In a large saucepan, warm the olive oil over medium-high heat.
2. Add the bell pepper, onions, and garlic and sauté until softened, about 4 minutes. Stir in the chili powder and paprika and sauté 1 minute.
3. Stir in the black beans, lentils, edamame, tomatoes, and corn and lower the heat to medium. Cook, stirring occasionally, until the chili is hot and fragrant, about 25 minutes.
4. Serve topped with avocado.

Nutrition Info:

- Per Serving: Calories: 512 ; Fat: 16 g ;Saturated fat: 2 g ;Sodium: 105 mg

Pinto Bean Tortillas

Servings: 4

Cooking Time: 25 Min

Ingredients:

- 1 (15 oz) can low-sodium pinto beans, rinsed and drained
- ¼ cup canned fire-roasted tomato salsa
- ¾ cup dairy-free cheddar cheese, shredded and divided
- 1 medium red bell pepper, seeded, chopped and divided
- 2 tbsp. olive oil, divided
- 4 large, wholegrain tortillas

Directions:

1. Place the drained pinto beans and the tomato salsa together in a food processor. Process until smooth.
2. Spread ½ cup of the pinto bean mixture on each tortilla. Sprinkle each tortilla with 3 tbsp. of dairy-free cheddar cheese and ¼ cup of red bell pepper. Fold in half and repeat with the remaining tortillas.
3. Add 1 tbsp. of olive oil to a large, heavy-bottom pan over medium heat until hot. Place the first two folded tortillas in the pan. Cover and cook for 2 minutes until the tortillas are crispy on the bottom. Flip and cook for 2 minutes until crispy on the other side.
4. Repeat with the remaining folded tortillas and the remaining olive oil. Keep warm until ready to serve.

Nutrition Info:

- Per Serving: Calories:438 ; Fat: 21 g ;Saturated fat: 5 g ;Sodium: 561 mg

Sour-cream-and-herb Omelet

Servings: 4

Cooking Time: X

Ingredients:

- 1 tablespoon olive oil
- 2 shallots, minced
- 1 clove garlic, minced
- 2 cups egg substitute
- ¼ cup skim milk
- ¼ cup low-fat sour cream 1 teaspoon grated lemon zest
- 1 teaspoon fresh thyme leaves
- 1/8 teaspoon pepper
- 2/3 cup shredded extra-sharp Cheddar cheese

Directions:

1. In a large nonstick skillet, heat olive oil over medium heat. Add shallots and garlic; stir-fry for 2 minutes, until fragrant.
2. In medium bowl, combine egg substitute and milk and beat well. Add to saucepan; cook, running a spatula around the edges, and lifting the edges to let uncooked mixture flow underneath. Cook until eggs are set and bottom is golden brown, about 4–6 minutes.
3. Meanwhile, in small bowl combine sour cream, lemon zest, thyme, and pepper and mix well. Sprinkle omelet with Cheddar, cover pan, and remove from heat. Let stand for 3 minutes, then cut into pieces and serve with the sour-cream mixture.

Nutrition Info:

- Per Serving: Calories: 243.49; Fat:15.62 g ;Saturated fat: 6.42 g ;Sodium: 354.41 mg

Roasted Garlic Soufflé

Servings: 4

Cooking Time: X

Ingredients:

- 1 head Roasted Garlic
- 2 tablespoons olive oil
- 1 cup finely chopped cooked turkey breast
- ¼ cup grated Parmesan cheese
- 1/8 teaspoon pepper
- 1 egg
- ¼ cup low-fat sour cream
- 6 egg whites
- ¼ teaspoon cream of tartar
- ¼ cup chopped flat-leaf parsley

Directions:

1. Preheat oven to 375ºF. Grease the bottom of a 2-quart soufflé dish with peanut oil and set aside. Squeeze the garlic from the papery skins. Discard skins, and in medium bowl, combine olive oil with the garlic. Add turkey, cheese, pepper, egg, and sour cream, and mix well.
2. In large bowl, combine egg whites with cream of tartar. Beat until stiff peaks form. Stir a spoonful of egg whites into the turkey mixture and stir well. Then fold in remaining egg whites. Fold in parsley.
3. Spoon mixture into prepared soufflé dish. Bake for 40–50 minutes or until the soufflé is puffed and golden. Serve immediately.

Nutrition Info:

- Per Serving: Calories:223.79 ; Fat: 14.23 g ;Saturated fat:3.92 g ;Sodium: 253.37 mg

Garbanzo Sandwich

Servings: 4

Cooking Time: 10 Min

Ingredients:

- 1 (15 oz) can low-sodium garbanzo bean, drained and rinsed
- ¼ cup medium red onion, finely chopped
- ¼ cup plain unsweetened coconut milk yoghurt
- 1½ tsp whole-grain mustard
- Himalayan pink salt
- Ground black pepper
- 2 green leaf lettuce leaves
- 4 whole-grain bread slices

Directions:

1. In a medium-sized mixing bowl, use a fork to mash up the garbanzo beans roughly. There must be some chunky pieces.
2. Add the red onion, coconut milk yoghurt, and wholegrain mustard. Season with salt and pepper to taste, mix to combine.
3. Place 1 green leaf lettuce leaf on each of the 2 wholegrain bread slices. Divide the garbanzo bean mixture between the 2 slices of bread on top of the lettuce leaf.
4. Top with the remaining slice of bread and serve.

Nutrition Info:

- Per Serving: Calories: 162; Fat: 3 g ;Saturated fat: 1 g ;Sodium: 287mg

Chopped Vegetable Tabbouleh

Servings: X

Cooking Time: X

Ingredients:

- 2 cups cooked quinoa
- 2 cup finely chopped cauliflower
- ½ cup shelled edamame
- 2 tomatoes, chopped
- ½ English cucumber, chopped
- 1 scallion, white and green parts, thinly sliced
- ¼ cup chopped fresh parsley
- 2 tablespoons chopped fresh mint
- Juice and zest of 1 lemon
- Sea salt
- Freshly ground black pepper

Directions:

1. In a medium bowl, toss together the quinoa, cauliflower, edamame, tomatoes, cucumber, scallions, parsley, mint, lemon juice, and lemon zest.
2. Season with salt and pepper.
3. Serve.

Nutrition Info:

- Per Serving: Calories: 430 ; Fat:8 g ;Saturated fat: 1 g ;Sodium: 58 mg

Peanut-butter-banana Skewered Sammies

Servings: 4–6

Cooking Time: X

Ingredients:

- ½ cup natural no-salt peanut butter
- 8 slices Honey-Wheat Sesame Bread
- 2 bananas
- 2 tablespoons lime juice
- 2 tablespoons butter or margarine, softened

Directions:

1. Spread peanut butter on one side of each slice of bread. Slice bananas, and as you work, sprinkle with lime juice. Make sandwiches by putting the bananas on the peanut butter and combining slices.
2. Butter the outsides of the sandwiches. Heat grill and cook sandwiches until bread is crisp and golden brown. Remove from grill, cut into quarters, and skewer on wood or metal skewers. Serve immediately.

Nutrition Info:

- Per Serving: Calories:376.36; Fat:18.67 g ;Saturated fat: 5.57 g ;Sodium: 77.44 mg

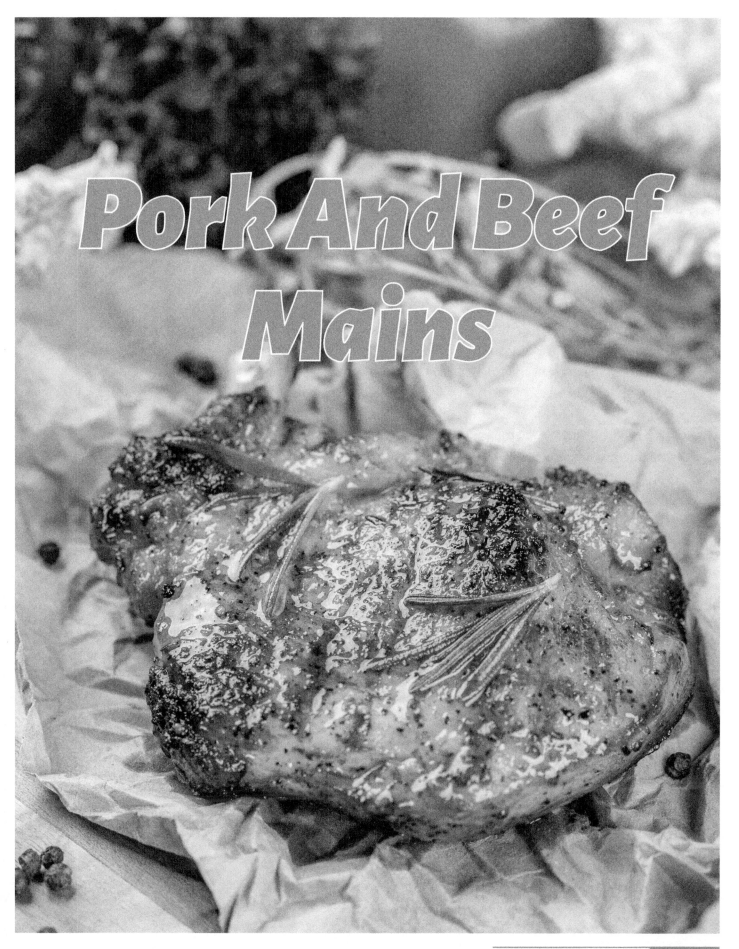

Pork And Beef Mains

Pork And Beef Mains

Pork Tenderloin With Orange Relish

Servings: X

Cooking Time: 25 Minutes

Ingredients:

- For the relish
- 1 large orange, chopped
- ½ red bell pepper, chopped
- ½ scallion, white and green parts, sliced thinly
- 1 tablespoon honey
- 1 teaspoon chopped jalapeño pepper
- ¼ teaspoon chopped fresh cilantro
- Pinch sea salt
- For the pork
- 1 (6-ounce) pork tenderloin, fat trimmed
- ¼ teaspoon ground coriander
- Sea salt
- Freshly ground black pepper
- 2 teaspoons olive oil

Directions:

1. To make the relish
2. In a small bowl, stir together the orange, bell pepper, scallions, honey, jalapeño, cilantro, and salt until well mixed.
3. Set aside.
4. To make the pork
5. Preheat the oven to 400°F.
6. Season the pork lightly with coriander, salt, and pepper.
7. In a medium oven-safe skillet, warm the oil over medium-high heat.
8. Add the pork and cook until browned on all sides, about 6 minutes.
9. Transfer the skillet to the oven and roast until the pork is just cooked through, 15 to 16 minutes.
10. Let the pork rest for 10 minutes, then slice against the grain into ½-inch slices.
11. Serve the pork topped with the relish.

Nutrition Info:

- Per Serving: Calories: 246 ; Fat: 8 g ;Saturated fat: 2 g ;Sodium: 202 mg

Simple Pork Burgers

Servings: X

Cooking Time: 15 Minutes

Ingredients:

- ½ pound extra-lean ground pork
- 1 large egg white
- 1 scallion, white parts only, chopped
- ¼ cup ground almonds
- ¼ teaspoon minced garlic
- ⅛ teaspoon allspice
- Sea salt
- Freshly ground black pepper

Directions:

1. Preheat a grill to medium-high heat.
2. In a medium bowl, thoroughly mix together the pork, egg white, scallion, almonds, garlic, and allspice. Season the mixture with salt and pepper.
3. Form the mixture into 2 burgers.
4. Place the burgers on the grill and cook until they are just cooked through, 7 to 8 minutes per side, depending on the thickness of the patties.
5. Serve with your favorite toppings.

Nutrition Info:

- Per Serving: Calories: 243 ; Fat: 13 g ;Saturated fat: 3 g ;Sodium: 83 mg

Pork Cutlets With Fennel And Kale

Servings: X

Cooking Time: 30 Minutes

Ingredients:

- 2 (4-ounce) boneless pork top-loin chops
- Sea salt
- Freshly ground black pepper
- 2 teaspoons olive oil, divided
- 1 small fennel bulb, thinly sliced
- ½ cup chopped sweet onion
- 1 teaspoon garlic
- ¼ cup white wine
- ¼ low-sodium chicken broth
- 2 cups shredded kale
- 2 teaspoons chopped fresh basil, for garnish

Directions:

1. Pound the pork chops to about ¼-inch thick between two sheets of parchment paper and season each with salt and pepper.
2. In a large skillet, heat 1 teaspoon olive oil over medium-high heat and sear the pork until lightly browned, about 4 minutes per side. Remove the pork and cover with foil to keep warm.
3. Add the remaining 1 teaspoon olive oil to the skillet and sauté the fennel, onions, and garlic until softened, 6 to 7 minutes.
4. Add the wine and chicken broth to the skillet and bring the liquid to a boil. Reduce the heat to low, then simmer until the liquid reduces by half, about 5 minutes.
5. Return the pork to the skillet and cook until the pork is tender, about 6 minutes.
6. Stir in the kale and simmer until the kale is wilted, about 4 more minutes.
7. Serve topped with basil.

Nutrition Info:

- Per Serving: Calories: 366 ; Fat: 20 g ;Saturated fat: 7 g ;Sodium: 264 mg

Dark Beer Beef Chili

Servings: X

Cooking Time: 50 Minutes

Ingredients:

- 1 teaspoon olive oil
- 6 ounces extra-lean ground beef
- ½ sweet onion, chopped
- 1 green bell pepper, diced
- 1 teaspoon minced garlic
- 2 cups low-sodium canned diced tomatoes, with their juices
- ½ cup low-sodium canned kidney beans, rinsed and drained
- ½ cup low-sodium canned lentils, rinsed and drained
- ½ cup dark beer
- 1 tablespoon chili powder
- ½ teaspoon ground cumin
- Pinch cayenne powder
- 2 teaspoons chopped fresh cilantro, for garnish
- 4 tablespoons fat-free sour cream, for garnish

Directions:

1. In a large saucepan, warm the oil over medium-high heat.
2. Add the ground beef and cook until browned, about 5 minutes.
3. Add the onions, bell pepper, and garlic and sauté until softened, about 4 minutes.
4. Stir in the tomatoes, kidney beans, lentils, beer, chili powder, cumin, and cayenne powder.
5. Bring the mixture to a boil and then reduce the heat. Simmer, partially covered, until the flavors come together and the liquid is almost gone, 35 to 40 minutes.
6. Serve topped with cilantro and sour cream.

Nutrition Info:

- Per Serving: Calories: 415 ; Fat: 10 g ;Saturated fat: 2 g ;Sodium: 125 mg

Stir-fried Crispy Orange Beef

Servings: 4

Cooking Time: 12 Minutes

Ingredients:

- ½ cup low-sodium beef broth, divided
- 3 tablespoons orange juice
- 1 teaspoon fresh orange zest
- 1 teaspoon low-sodium soy sauce
- 1 teaspoon Thai chili paste
- 2 tablespoons rice flour or cornstarch, divided
- ½ pound top round steak
- 1 teaspoon paprika
- ⅛ teaspoon cayenne pepper
- 1 teaspoon olive oil
- 3 scallions, chopped
- 2 cups snow pea pods
- 1 red bell pepper, seeded and chopped
- 1 carrot, grated

Directions:

1. In a small bowl, combine all but 1 tablespoon of the beef broth, the orange juice, orange zest, soy sauce, Thai chili paste, and 1 tablespoon of the rice flour or cornstarch, and mix well. Set aside.
2. Trim off the fat from the steak and discard. Slice into thin strips and put in a medium bowl. Add the remaining 1 tablespoon rice flour or cornstarch, the paprika, and cayenne pepper to the beef and toss to coat.
3. Heat ½ teaspoon of the olive oil in a nonstick skillet or wok over high heat.
4. Add half the beef strips in a single layer. Let them cook for 2 minutes, then turn and cook for 2 to 3 minutes or until the beef is crisp. Remove the beef to a clean plate.
5. Repeat with remaining ½ teaspoon olive oil and beef strips. Remove the beef to the plate.
6. Reduce the heat to medium high. Add reserved 1 tablespoon beef broth to the skillet, then add the scallions, pea pods, and carrots. Stir-fry for 2 to 3 minutes, or until the vegetables are crisp-tender.
7. Add the orange–beef broth mixture to the skillet and stir-fry for 1 to 2 minutes or until the sauce has thickened slightly. Add the beef strips, and stir-fry for 1 minute.

Nutrition Info:

- Per Serving: Calories: 175 ; Fat: 4 g ;Saturated fat: 1 g ;Sodium: 194 mg

Pork Skewers With Cherry Tomatoes

Servings: 4

Cooking Time: X

Ingredients:

- ¼ pound pork tenderloin, cubed
- 24 cherry tomatoes
- 1 onion, cut into eighths
- 2 tablespoons olive oil
- 1 tablespoon lemon juice
- 1/8 teaspoon pepper
- 2 tablespoons chopped flat-leaf parsley
- 1 tablespoon fresh oregano leaves
- ¼ cup shredded Parmesan cheese

Directions:

1. Prepare and preheat grill. Thread pork, cherry tomatoes, and onion on metal skewers. In small bowl, combine olive oil, lemon juice, pepper, parsley, and oregano leaves. Brush skewers with olive oil mixture.
2. Grill skewers 6″ from medium coals for 8–10 minutes, turning and brushing occasionally with marinade, until pork registers 155ºF. Sprinkle with Parmesan, let stand to melt, and serve.

Nutrition Info:

- Per Serving: Calories:240.01; Fat: 10.48 g ;Saturated fat: 3.50 g ;Sodium:177.18 mg

Lemon Garlic Flank Steak Wraps

Servings: 4

Cooking Time: 15 Minutes

Ingredients:

- ½ pound flank steak
- ⅛ teaspoon garlic powder
- Pinch salt
- ⅛ teaspoon lemon pepper
- 3 tablespoons fresh lemon juice
- 1 tablespoon orange juice
- 1 red bell pepper, seeded and sliced
- 1 cucumber, sliced
- 3 stalks celery, sliced
- 2 cups fresh baby spinach
- 4 (8-inch) whole-wheat flour tortillas

Directions:

1. In a shallow bowl, sprinkle the flank steak with the garlic powder, salt, and lemon pepper. Drizzle all over with the lemon juice and orange juice and let stand for 10 minutes while you prepare the rest of the ingredients.
2. Heat a grill pan or nonstick skillet over medium-high heat. Add the steak, and cook 5 to 6 minutes per side, turning once, until cooked to at least 145°F on a meat thermometer.
3. Remove the steak from the grill and let rest for 2 minutes. Cut the steak across the grain into thin slices.
4. Divide the steak, vegetables, and spinach, among the 4 tortillas. Roll up, tucking in the ends, cut in half, and serve.

Nutrition Info:

- Per Serving: Calories: 292 ; Fat: 9 g ;Saturated fat: 4 g ;Sodium: 513 mg

Fruit-stuffed Pork Tenderloin

Servings: 6

Cooking Time: X

Ingredients:

- 1½ pounds pork tenderloin
- ¼ cup dry white wine
- 6 prunes, chopped
- 5 dried apricots, chopped
- 1 onion, chopped
- 2 tablespoons flour
- 1/8 teaspoon salt
- 1/8 teaspoon pepper
- 2 tablespoons olive oil
- ½ cup Low-Sodium Chicken Broth
- 1 teaspoon dried thyme leaves

Directions:

1. Trim excess fat from meat. Cut tenderloin lengthwise, cutting to, but not through, the other side. Open up the meat and place on work surface, cut side up. Lightly pound with a rolling pin or meat mallet until about ½" thick.
2. In small saucepan, combine wine, prunes, apricots, and onion. Simmer for 10 minutes or until fruit is soft and wine is absorbed. Place this mixture in the center of the pork tenderloin. Roll the pork around the fruit mixture, using a toothpick to secure.
3. Sprinkle pork with flour, salt, and pepper. In ovenproof saucepan, heat olive oil. Add pork; brown on all sides, turning frequently, about 5–6 minutes. Add broth and thyme to saucepan. Bake for 25–35 minutes or until internal temperature registers 155ºF. Let pork stand for 5 minutes, remove toothpicks, and slice to serve.

Nutrition Info:

- Per Serving: Calories: 249.06 ; Fat: 9.82 g ;Saturated fat: 2.41 g ;Sodium: 102.85 mg

Pan-seared Beef Tenderloin With Wild Mushrooms

Servings: X

Cooking Time: 25 Minutes

Ingredients:

- 2 (4-ounce) beef tenderloin steaks, fat trimmed
- Sea salt
- Freshly ground black pepper
- Nonstick olive oil cooking spray
- 1 tablespoon canola oil
- 1 teaspoon minced garlic
- 4 cups thinly sliced wild mushrooms (shiitake, oyster, portobello, and chanterelles)
- ½ teaspoon chopped fresh thyme

Directions:

1. Season the steaks lightly with salt and pepper.
2. Lightly coat a large skillet with cooking spray and place it over medium heat. Sear the steaks until they reach your desired doneness, 5 minutes per side for medium.
3. Remove the steaks and set aside.
4. Add the canola oil to the skillet and sauté the garlic until softened, about 3 minutes.
5. Add the mushrooms and cook, stirring occasionally, until lightly caramelized, 7 to 8 minutes.
6. Stir in the thyme and season with salt and pepper.
7. Serve the steaks with the mushrooms.

Nutrition Info:

- Per Serving: Calories: 267 ; Fat: 15 g ;Saturated fat: 3 g ;Sodium: 72 mg

Cabbage Roll Sauté

Servings: X

Cooking Time: 30 Minutes

Ingredients:

- 4 cups water
- ½ cup brown rice, rinsed
- Nonstick olive oil cooking spray
- 6 ounces extra-lean ground beef
- ¼ small sweet onion, chopped
- ½ teaspoon minced garlic
- 2 cups crushed tomatoes
- 1 tablespoon brown sugar
- 2 teaspoons balsamic vinegar
- ¼ teaspoon paprika
- 2 cups thinly shredded cabbage
- 2 teaspoons chopped fresh parsley, for garnish

Directions:

1. Warm the water in a medium saucepan over high heat and bring to a boil.
2. Add the rice and reduce the heat to medium-low. Simmer until the rice is tender, about 30 minutes.
3. Drain any excess water and set the rice aside, covered, to keep warm.
4. Generously coat a large skillet with cooking spray and place over medium-high heat.
5. Add the beef and cook until browned, breaking it up, 5 to 7 minutes.
6. Stir in the onion and garlic and sauté until the vegetables are softened, about 3 minutes.
7. Stir in the crushed tomatoes, sugar, vinegar, and paprika and bring the sauce to a boil.
8. Stir in the cabbage and reduce the heat to low. Simmer until the cabbage is very tender, 10 to 12 minutes.
9. Serve the cabbage roll mixture over the rice, topped with parsley.

Nutrition Info:

- Per Serving: Calories: 473 ; Fat: 9 g ;Saturated fat: 3 g ;Sodium: 328 mg

Pork Goulash

Servings: 4

Cooking Time: 15 Minutes

Ingredients:

- ½ pound lean ground pork
- 2 onions, chopped
- 8 ounces sliced button mushrooms
- 4 cloves garlic, minced
- 3 stalks celery, sliced
- ½ cup grated carrot
- 2 teaspoons smoked paprika
- Pinch salt
- ⅛ teaspoon white pepper
- 1 (14-ounce) can no-salt-added diced tomatoes
- 1 (8-ounce) can no-salt-added tomato sauce
- 2 tablespoons tomato paste
- ½ cup water
- 1 cup whole-wheat orzo

Directions:

1. In a large skillet over medium-high, sauté the pork, onions, mushrooms, garlic, celery, and carrot for 4 minutes, stirring to break up the pork, until the meat is almost cooked through.
2. Add the paprika, salt, white pepper, tomatoes, tomato sauce, tomato paste, and water, and bring to a simmer. Simmer for 1 minute.
3. Add the orzo to the skillet and stir, making sure that the pasta is covered by liquid. Simmer for 10 to 12 minutes or until the pasta is cooked al dente. Serve immediately.

Nutrition Info:

- Per Serving: Calories:299 ; Fat:7 g ;Saturated fat: 2 g ;Sodium: 128 mg

Pepper Pot

Servings: 4

Cooking Time: 15 Minutes

Ingredients:

- ¾ pound boneless center cut pork chops
- ⅛ teaspoon cayenne pepper
- 1 teaspoon olive oil
- 1 onion, chopped
- 4 cloves garlic, minced
- 1 red bell pepper, seeded and chopped
- 1 yellow bell pepper, seeded and chopped
- 2 Yukon Gold potatoes, diced
- 2 jalapeño pepper, seeded and minced
- 1 red Thai chile pepper, minced (optional)
- 1 (14-ounce) can no-salt-added diced tomatoes
- 1 cup low-sodium chicken broth
- 1 teaspoon Thai garlic chili paste (optional)
- 1 teaspoon ground cinnamon

Directions:

1. Trim excess fat off the pork chops and cut the meat into 1-inch pieces. Sprinkle with the cayenne pepper.
2. Heat the olive oil in a large nonstick skillet over medium heat. Add the pork, onion, and garlic, and sauté 3 to 4 minutes or until the pork is lightly browned.
3. Add the red bell pepper, yellow bell pepper, potato, jalapeño, Thai chile pepper (if using), tomatoes, chicken broth, chili paste (if using), and cinnamon, and bring to a simmer. Reduce the heat to medium-low and simmer 10 to 12 minutes, or until the potato is tender and the sauce is slightly thickened. Serve immediately.

Nutrition Info:

- Per Serving: Calories: 258 ; Fat: 6 g ;Saturated fat: 1 g ;Sodium: 104 mg

Pork And Fennel Stir Fry

Servings: 4

Cooking Time: 10 Minutes

Ingredients:

- 1 fennel bulb
- 1½ cups low-sodium chicken broth
- 1 tablespoon rice wine vinegar
- 1 tablespoon honey
- 2 tablespoons cornstarch
- 1 teaspoon soy sauce
- 12 ounces boneless top loin pork chops
- Pinch salt
- ⅛ teaspoon white pepper
- 2 teaspoons olive oil
- 8 ounces cremini mushrooms, sliced
- 3 stalks celery, sliced
- 2 cloves garlic, minced

Directions:

1. To prepare the fennel, trim the root end and cut off the stalk. Cut the bulb in half and peel off the outer skin. Slice the fennel thinly crosswise, and set aside. Finely slice the stalks, if desired. Cut some of the fennel fronds into tiny pieces with kitchen scissors, and set aside.
2. In a small bowl, combine the chicken broth, rice wine vinegar, honey, cornstarch, and soy sauce, and whisk to combine. Set aside.
3. Trim excess fat from the pork chops, and cut into 1-inch pieces. Sprinkle with the salt and white pepper.
4. Heat the olive oil in a large nonstick skillet or wok over medium-high heat. Add the pork and stir-fry until lightly browned, about 3 minutes. Remove the pork to a clean plate.
5. Add the fennel, fennel stalks if using, mushrooms, celery, and garlic to the skillet, and stir-fry for 3 to 4 minutes or until crisp-tender.
6. Stir the broth mixture, add it to the skillet, and bring to a simmer.
7. Add the pork and stir-fry 2 to 3 minutes or until the pork is cooked to at least 150°F on a meat thermometer and the sauce is thickened. Sprinkle with the reserved fennel fronds and serve immediately.

Nutrition Info:

- Per Serving: Calories: 204 ; Fat: 7 g ;Saturated fat: 2 g ;Sodium: 324 mg

Mustard Pork Tenderloin

Servings: 6

Cooking Time: X

Ingredients:

- 2 tablespoons red wine
- 1 tablespoon sugar
- 1 tablespoon olive oil
- 1¼ pounds pork tenderloin
- ¼ cup low-fat sour cream
- 3 tablespoons Dijon mustard
- 1 tablespoon minced fresh chives

Directions:

1. In glass baking dish, combine red wine, sugar, and olive oil. Add pork tenderloin; turn to coat. Cover and refrigerate for 8 hours.
2. Preheat oven to 325ºF. Let pork stand at room temperature for 20 minutes. Roast for 30 minutes, basting occasionally with the marinade.
3. In small bowl, combine sour cream, mustard, and chives. Spread over the tenderloin. Continue roasting for 25–35 minutes or until pork registers 160ºF. Let stand for 5 minutes, then slice to serve.

Nutrition Info:

- Per Serving: Calories: 209.84 ; Fat:9.08 g ;Saturated fat: 2.98 g ;Sodium: 147.13 mg

Cowboy Steak With Chimichurri Sauce

Servings: 4–6

Cooking Time: X

Ingredients:

- 1 cup chopped parsley
- ¼ cup minced fresh oregano leaves
- ¼ cup extra-virgin olive oil
- 2 tablespoons lemon juice
- 3 tablespoons sherry vinegar
- 6 cloves garlic, minced
- 1/8 teaspoon salt
- ¼ teaspoon pepper
- 1 pound flank steak
- 2 tablespoons red wine
- 2 tablespoons olive oil

Directions:

1. In blender or food processor, combine parsley, oregano, olive oil, lemon juice, sherry vinegar, garlic, salt, and pepper; blend or process until smooth. Pour into small bowl, cover, and refrigerate until ready to use.
2. Pierce flank steak all over with a fork. Place in large heavy-duty zip-close freezer bag and add red wine and olive oil. Seal bag and squish to mix. Place in pan and refrigerate for 8–12 hours.
3. When ready to eat, prepare and preheat grill. Grill steak for 6–10 minutes, turning once, until desired doneness. Remove from grill and let stand, covered, for 10 minutes. Slice thinly against the grain and serve with the Chimichurri Sauce.

Nutrition Info:

- Per Serving: Calories:244.50; Fat:18.59 g ;Saturated fat: 5.20 g ;Sodium: 117.31 mg

Sirloin Steak With Root Vegetables

Servings: X

Cooking Time: 40 Minutes

Ingredients:

- 1 (10-ounce) sirloin steak, fat trimmed
- Sea salt
- Freshly ground black pepper
- 2 carrots, cut into 1-inch chunks
- 2 parsnip, cut into 1-inch chunks
- 1 small celeriac, peeled and cut into 1-inch chunks
- 1 small sweet potato, peeled and cut into 1-inch chunks
- 6 beets, peeled and halved
- 1 tablespoon olive oil, plus extra for drizzling

Directions:

1. Preheat the oven to 400°F.
2. Line a sheet pan with foil and set aside.
3. Season the steak with salt and pepper and set aside.
4. Spread the veggies on the sheet pan, leaving room for the steak. Season them lightly with salt and pepper and drizzle with 1 tablespoon olive oil.
5. Roast the veggies until they are lightly caramelized and tender, about 30 minutes.
6. Remove the sheet pan from the oven and add the steak.
7. Increase the oven temperature to broil.
8. Place the sheet pan into the oven and broil until the steak is browned, 4 to 5 minutes per side for medium-rare, or until it reaches your desired doneness.
9. Serve.

Nutrition Info:

- Per Serving: Calories: 565 ; Fat: 26 g ;Saturated fat: 8 g ;Sodium: 274 mg

Steak With Mushroom Sauce

Servings: 6

Cooking Time: X

Ingredients:

- 1 to 1¼ pounds flank steak
- 2 tablespoons red wine
- 1 tablespoon olive oil
- 1 tablespoon butter
- 1 onion, minced
- 1 (8-ounce) package sliced mushrooms
- 2 tablespoons flour
- 1½ cups Low-Sodium Beef Broth
- ¼ teaspoon ground coriander
- 2 teaspoons Worcestershire sauce
- 1/8 teaspoon pepper

Directions:

1. In glass dish, combine flank steak, red wine, and olive oil. Cover and marinate for at least 8 hours.
2. When ready to eat, prepare and preheat grill. Drain steak, reserving marinade.
3. In large skillet, melt butter over medium heat. Add onion and mushrooms; cook and stir until liquid evaporates, about 8–9 minutes. Stir in flour; cook and stir for 2 minutes. Add beef broth and marinade from beef and bring to a boil. Stir in coriander, Worcestershire sauce, and pepper; reduce heat to low and simmer while cooking steak.
4. Cook steak 6″ from medium coals for 7–10 minutes, turning once, until steak reaches desired doneness. Remove from heat, cover, and let stand for 10 minutes. Slice thinly against the grain and serve with mushroom sauce.

Nutrition Info:

- Per Serving: Calories: 262.45; Fat: 16.09 g ;Saturated fat: 6.42 g;Sodium: 114.22 mg

Prosciutto Fruit Omelet

Servings: 4

Cooking Time: X

Ingredients:

- ¼ pound thinly sliced prosciutto
- ½ cup shredded part-skim mozzarella cheese
- 2 tablespoons grated Parmesan cheese
- 1 egg
- 8 egg whites
- ¼ cup low-fat sour cream
- 1/8 teaspoon pepper
- 1 tablespoon olive oil
- 1 apple, chopped

Directions:

1. Trim off excess fat from prosciutto and discard. Thinly slice the pro-sciutto and combine with the mozzarella and Parmesan cheeses. Set aside.
2. In large bowl, combine egg, egg whites, sour cream, and pepper and mix well. In large nonstick saucepan, heat olive oil over medium heat; add apples and stir until apples are tender. Pour in egg mixture.
3. Cook, running spatula around edges to let uncooked mixture flow underneath, until eggs are almost set and bottom is golden brown.
4. Sprinkle with cheese and ham mixture and cook for 2–3 minutes longer. Cover, remove from heat, and let stand for 2 minutes. Fold omelet over on itself and slide onto plate to serve.

Nutrition Info:

- Per Serving: Calories:221.48; Fat:12.35 g ;Saturated fat:4.99 g ;Sodium: 551.41 mg

Filet Mignon With Vegetables

Servings: 8–10

Cooking Time: X

Ingredients:

- 1 (16-ounce) package baby carrots, halved lengthwise
- 1 (8-ounce) package frozen pearl onions
- 16 new potatoes, halved
- 2 tablespoons olive oil
- 2 pounds filet mignon
- 1/8 teaspoon salt
- 1/8 teaspoon white pepper
- ½ cup dry red wine

Directions:

1. Preheat oven to 425ºF. Place carrots, onions, and potatoes in large roasting pan and drizzle with olive oil; toss to coat. Spread in an even layer. Roast for 15 minutes, then remove from oven.
2. Top with filet mignon; sprinkle the meat with salt and pepper. Pour wine over meat and vegetables.
3. Return to oven; roast for 20–30 minutes longer until beef registers 150ºF for medium. Remove from oven, tent with foil, and let stand for 5 minutes, then carve to serve.

Nutrition Info:

- Per Serving: Calories:442.64 ; Fat:11.83 g ;Saturated fat:3.77 g ;Sodium:140.70 mg

Classic Spaghetti And Meatballs

Servings: X

Cooking Time: 20 Minutes

Ingredients:

- Nonstick olive oil cooking spray
- 6 ounces extra-lean ground beef
- 1 large egg white
- ¼ cup ground almonds
- 2 teaspoons chopped fresh parsley
- ¼ teaspoon garlic powder
- Pinch sea salt
- Pinch freshly ground black pepper
- 2 cups Double Tomato Sauce or your favorite low-sodium marinara sauce
- 4 ounces dry spaghetti

Directions:

1. Preheat the oven to 400°F.
2. Line a baking sheet with parchment paper and spray it lightly with cooking spray. Set aside.
3. In a medium bowl, combine the ground beef, egg white, almonds, parsley, garlic powder, salt, and pepper until well mixed. Form the meat mixture into 12 meatballs and spread out on the baking sheet.
4. Bake the meatballs until cooked through, about 20 minutes. Remove from the oven and set aside.
5. While the meatballs are cooking, warm the sauce in a medium saucepan over medium heat. Cook the spaghetti according to package instructions.
6. Drain the pasta and serve topped with sauce and meatballs.

Nutrition Info:

- Per Serving: Calories: 574 ; Fat: 12 g ;Saturated fat: 2 g ;Sodium: 443 mg

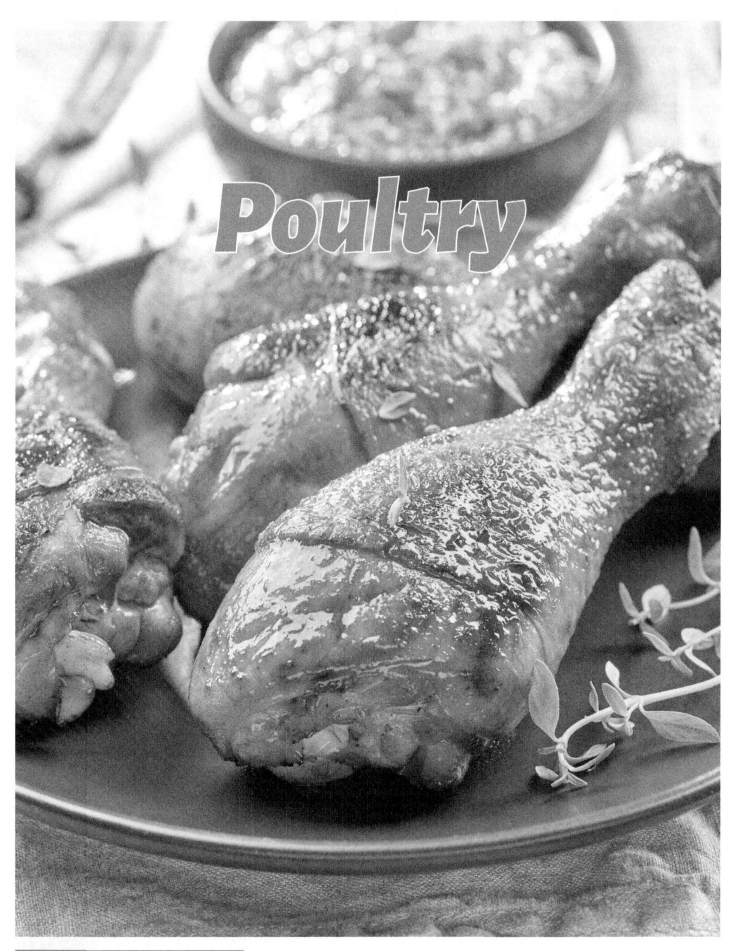

Poultry

Poultry

Turkey Oat Patties

Servings: 6

Cooking Time: 30 Min

Ingredients:

- Aluminum foil
- 1 lb. lean ground turkey
- ½ cup rolled oats
- ¼ cup sun-dried tomatoes julienne cut, drained
- ¼ cup brown onion, finely chopped
- ¼ cup parsley, finely chopped
- 1 tbsp. garlic, crushed
- 6 whole-wheat hamburger buns
- 1 ripe avocado, peeled, pitted, and mashed
- 6 iceberg lettuce leaves
- 6 Roma tomato slices
- Hamburger dill pickle chips

Directions:

1. Preheat the oven to broil. Line a baking sheet with aluminum foil.
2. In a large-sized mixing bowl, add the turkey, oats, sun-dried tomatoes, onion, parsley, and garlic, mix to combine. Shape into 6 patties.
3. Place the turkey patties on the baking sheet, and broil for 3 to 4 minutes on each side, until fully cooked and the juices run clear.
4. Meanwhile, prepare a self-serving platter with the buns, mashed avocado, lettuce leaves, tomato slices, and the dill pickle chips. Assemble the way you like.

Nutrition Info:

- Per Serving: Calories: 366 ; Fat: 15g;Saturated fat: 3 g ;Sodium: 52 mg

Mustard-roasted Almond Chicken Tenders

Servings: 4

Cooking Time: 15 Minutes

Ingredients:

- ¼ cup low-sodium yellow mustard
- 2 teaspoons yellow mustard seed
- ¼ teaspoon dry mustard
- ⅛ teaspoon garlic powder
- 1 egg white
- 2 tablespoons fresh lemon juice
- ¼ cup almond flour
- ¼ cup ground almonds
- 1 pound chicken tenders

Directions:

1. Preheat the oven to 400°F. Place a wire rack on a baking sheet.
2. In a shallow bowl, combine the yellow mustard, mustard seed, ground mustard, garlic powder, egg white, and lemon juice, and whisk well.
3. To a plate or shallow bowl, add the almond flour and ground almonds, and combine.
4. Dip the chicken tenders into the mustard-egg mixture, then into the almond mixture to coat. Place each tender on the rack on the baking pan as you work.
5. Bake the chicken for 12 to 15 minutes or until a meat thermometer registers 165°F. Serve immediately.

Nutrition Info:

- Per Serving: Calories: 166 ; Fat : 4 g ;Saturated fat: 0 g ;Sodium: 264 mg

Turkey Cutlets Parmesan

Servings: 6

Cooking Time: X

Ingredients:

- 1 egg white
- ¼ cup dry breadcrumbs
- 1/8 teaspoon pepper
- 4 tablespoons grated Parmesan cheese, divided
- 6 (4-ounce) turkey cutlets
- 2 tablespoons olive oil
- 1 (15-ounce) can no-salt tomato sauce
- 1 teaspoon dried Italian seasoning
- ½ cup finely shredded part-skim mozzarella cheese

Directions:

1. Preheat oven to 350ºF. Spray a 2-quart baking dish with nonstick cooking spray and set aside.
2. In shallow bowl, beat egg white until foamy. On plate, combine breadcrumbs, pepper, and 2 tablespoons Parmesan. Dip the turkey cutlets into the egg white, then into the breadcrumb mixture, turning to coat.
3. In large saucepan, heat olive oil over medium heat. Add turkey cutlets; brown on both sides, about 2–3 minutes per side. Place in prepared baking dish. Add tomato sauce and Italian seasoning to saucepan; bring to a boil.
4. Pour sauce over cutlets in baking pan and top with mozzarella cheese and remaining 2 tablespoons Parmesan. Bake for 25–35 minutes or until sauce bubbles and cheese melts and begins to brown. Serve with pasta, if desired.

Nutrition Info:

- Per Serving: Calories: 275.49; Fat: 10.98 g ;Saturated fat:3.43 g ;Sodium: 229.86 mg

Lemon Tarragon Turkey Medallions

Servings: 4

Cooking Time: 10 Minutes

Ingredients:

- 1 pound turkey tenderloin
- Pinch salt
- ⅛ teaspoon lemon pepper
- 2 tablespoons cornstarch
- 1 teaspoon dried tarragon leaves
- ¼ cup fresh lemon juice
- ½ cup low-sodium chicken stock
- 1 teaspoon grated fresh lemon zest
- 2 teaspoons olive oil

Directions:

1. Cut the turkey tenderloin crosswise into ½-inch slices. Sprinkle with the salt and lemon pepper.
2. In a small bowl, combine the cornstarch, tarragon, lemon juice, chicken stock, and lemon zest, and mix well.
3. Heat the olive oil in a large nonstick skillet over medium heat.
4. Add the turkey tenderloins. Cook for 2 minutes, and then turn and cook for another 2 minutes.
5. Add the lemon juice mixture to the skillet. Cook, stirring frequently, until the sauce boils and thickens and the turkey is cooked to 165°F on a meat thermometer. Serve immediately.

Nutrition Info:

- Per Serving: Calories: 169 ; Fat :3 g ;Saturated fat: 1 g ;Sodium: 77 mg

Hawaiian Chicken Stir-fry

Servings: 4

Cooking Time: 10 Minutes

Ingredients:

- 1 (8-ounce) can crushed pineapple, undrained
- ⅓ cup water
- 2 tablespoons cornstarch
- 1 teaspoon brown sugar
- 1 teaspoon low-sodium tamari sauce
- ¼ teaspoon ground ginger
- ⅛ teaspoon cayenne pepper
- 2 tablespoons unsweetened shredded coconut
- 2 tablespoons chopped macadamia nuts
- 2 teaspoons olive oil
- 1 onion, chopped
- 1 red bell pepper, seeded and chopped
- 3 (6-ounce) boneless, skinless chicken breasts, cubed

Directions:

1. In a medium bowl, combine the pineapple, water, cornstarch, brown sugar, tamari, ginger, and cayenne pepper, and mix well. Set aside.
2. Place a large nonstick skillet or wok over medium heat. Add the coconut and macadamia nuts, and toast for 1 to 2 minutes, stirring constantly, until fragrant. Remove from the skillet and set aside.
3. Add the olive oil to the skillet and heat over medium-high heat. Add the onion and red bell pepper, and stir-fry for 2 to 3 minutes or until almost tender.
4. Add the chicken to the wok, and stir-fry for 3 to 4 minutes or until lightly browned.
5. Stir the sauce, add to the skillet, and stir fry for 1 to 2 minutes longer until the sauce thickens and the chicken registers at 165°F when tested with a meat thermometer.
6. Serve immediately, topped with the toasted coconut and macadamia nuts.

Nutrition Info:

- Per Serving: Calories: 301 ; Fat : 12 g ;Saturated fat: 4 g ;Sodium: 131 mg

Chicken Breasts With New Potatoes

Servings: 6

Cooking Time: X

Ingredients:

- 12 small new red potatoes
- 2 tablespoons olive oil
- 1/8 teaspoon white pepper
- 4 cloves garlic, minced
- 1 teaspoon dried oregano leaves
- 2 tablespoons Dijon mustard
- 4 (4-ounce) boneless, skinless chicken breasts
- 1 cup cherry tomatoes

Directions:

1. Preheat oven to 400°F. Line a roasting pan with parchment paper and set aside. Scrub potatoes and cut each in half. Place in prepared pan.
2. In small bowl, combine oil, pepper, garlic, oregano, and mustard and mix well. Drizzle half of this mixture over the potatoes and toss to coat. Roast for 20 minutes.
3. Cut chicken breasts into quarters. Remove pan from oven and add chicken to potato mixture. Using a spatula, mix potatoes and chicken together. Drizzle with remaining oil mixture. Return to oven and roast for 15 minutes longer.
4. Add tomatoes to pan. Roast for 5–10 minutes longer, or until potatoes are tender and browned and chicken is thoroughly cooked.

Nutrition Info:

- Per Serving: Calories: 395.92; Fat: 9.57 g ;Saturated fat: 1.85 g;Sodium: 142.98 mg

Moroccan Chicken

Servings: 4

Cooking Time: 15 Minutes

Ingredients:

- 3 (4-ounce) boneless, skinless chicken thighs, cubed
- 1 teaspoon smoked paprika
- ½ teaspoon ground cinnamon
- ½ teaspoon ground cumin
- ⅛ teaspoon ground ginger
- 1 cup low-sodium chicken broth
- 2 tablespoons fresh lemon juice
- 1 tablespoon cornstarch
- 1 teaspoon olive oil
- 1 onion, chopped
- 3 cloves garlic, minced
- 2 cups sugar snap peas
- 1 cup shredded carrots

Directions:

1. Put the cubed chicken in a medium bowl. Sprinkle with the paprika, cinnamon, cumin, and ginger, and work the spices into the meat. Set aside.
2. In a small bowl, combine the chicken broth, lemon juice, and cornstarch and mix well. Set aside.
3. Heat the olive oil in a large nonstick skillet over medium-high heat. Add the chicken thighs, and sauté for 5 minutes or until the chicken starts to brown. Remove the chicken from the pan and set aside.
4. Add the onion and garlic to the skillet, and sauté for 3 minutes.
5. Add the sugar snap peas and carrots to the skillet and sauté for 2 minutes.
6. Return the chicken to the skillet and stir. Add the chicken broth mixture, bring to a simmer, and turn down the heat to low. Simmer 3 to 4 minutes or until the sauce thickens, the vegetables are tender, and the chicken is cooked to 165°F on a meat thermometer.

Serve hot.

Nutrition Info:

- Per Serving: Calories: 165 ; Fat : 5 g ;Saturated fat: 1 g ;Sodium: 112 mg

Italian Chicken Bake

Servings: 4

Cooking Time: 25 Min

Ingredients:

- 1 lb. chicken breasts, halved lengthwise into 4 pieces
- ½ tsp garlic powder
- ½ tsp fine sea salt
- ¼ tsp ground black pepper
- ¼ tsp Italian seasoning
- ½ cup basil, finely chopped
- 4 part-skim mozzarella cheese slices
- 2 large Roma tomatoes, finely chopped

Directions:

1. Heat the oven to 400°F gas mark 6.
2. Season the cut chicken breasts with garlic powder, salt, pepper and Italian seasoning.
3. Place the seasoned chicken breasts on a baking sheet. Bake for 18 to 22 minutes, or until the chicken breasts are cooked through. Remove from the oven and set it to broil on high.
4. Evenly place the basil, 1 mozzarella slice and tomatoes on each chicken breast.
5. Return the baking sheet to the oven and broil for 2 to 3 minutes, until the cheese has melted and browned.
6. Remove from the oven and serve hot.

Nutrition Info:

- Per Serving: Calories: 239 ; Fat: 9 g ;Saturated fat: 4 g ;Sodium: 524 mg

Asian Chicken Stir-fry

Servings: 4

Cooking Time: X

Ingredients:

- 2 (5-ounce) boneless, skinless chicken breasts
- ½ cup Low-Sodium Chicken Broth
- 1 tablespoon low-sodium soy sauce
- 1 tablespoon cornstarch
- 1 tablespoon sherry
- 2 tablespoons peanut oil
- 1 onion, sliced
- 3 cloves garlic, minced
- 1 tablespoon grated ginger root
- 1 cup snow peas
- ½ cup canned sliced water chestnuts, drained
- 1 yellow summer squash, sliced
- ¼ cup chopped unsalted peanuts

Directions:

1. Cut chicken into strips and set aside. In small bowl, combine chicken broth, soy sauce, cornstarch, and sherry and set aside.
2. In large skillet or wok, heat peanut oil over medium-high heat. Add chicken; stir-fry until almost cooked, about 3–4 minutes. Remove to plate. Add onion, garlic, and ginger root to skillet; stir-fry for 4 minutes longer. Then add snow peas, water chestnuts, and squash; stir-fry for 2 minutes longer.
3. Stir chicken broth mixture and add to skillet along with chicken. Stir-fry for 3–4 minutes longer or until chicken is thoroughly cooked and sauce is thickened and bubbly. Sprinkle with peanuts and serve immediately.

Nutrition Info:

- Per Serving: Calories: 252.42; Fat: 12.42 g ;Saturated fat:2.06 g ;Sodium: 202.04 mg

Sautéed Chicken With Roasted Garlic Sauce

Servings: 4

Cooking Time: X

Ingredients:

- 1 head Roasted Garlic
- 1/3 cup Low-Sodium Chicken Broth
- ½ teaspoon dried oregano leaves
- 4 (4-ounce) boneless, skinless chicken breasts
- ¼ cup flour
- 1/8 teaspoon salt
- 1/8 teaspoon pepper
- ¼ teaspoon paprika
- 2 tablespoons olive oil

Directions:

1. Squeeze garlic cloves from the skins and combine in small saucepan with chicken broth and oregano leaves.
2. On shallow plate, combine flour, salt, pepper, and paprika. Dip chicken into this mixture to coat.
3. In large skillet, heat 2 tablespoons olive oil. At the same time, place the saucepan with the garlic mixture over medium heat. Add the chicken to the hot olive oil; cook for 5 minutes without moving. Then carefully turn chicken and cook for 4–7 minutes longer until chicken is thoroughly cooked.
4. Stir garlic sauce with wire whisk until blended. Serve with the chicken.

Nutrition Info:

- Per Serving: Calories: 267.01; Fat: 7.78g ;Saturated fat:1.65 g ;Sodium: 158.61 mg

Texas Bbq Chicken Thighs

Servings: 6

Cooking Time: X

Ingredients:

- 2 tablespoons olive oil
- 1 onion, chopped
- 4 cloves garlic, minced
- 1 jalapeño pepper, minced
- ¼ cup orange juice
- 1 tablespoon low-sodium soy sauce
- 2 tablespoons apple-cider vinegar
- 2 tablespoons brown sugar
- 2 tablespoons Dijon mustard
- 1 (14-ounce) can crushed tomatoes, undrained
- ½ teaspoon cumin
- 1 tablespoon chili powder
- ¼ teaspoon pepper
- 6 (4-ounce) boneless, skinless chicken thighs
- 3 tablespoons cornstarch
- ¼ cup water

Directions:

1. In a small skillet, heat olive oil over medium heat. Add onion and garlic; cook and stir until crisp-tender, about 4 minutes. Place in 3–4 quart slow cooker and add jalapeño, orange juice, soy sauce, vinegar, brown sugar, mustard, tomatoes, cumin, chili powder, and pepper.
2. Add chicken to the sauce, pushing chicken into the sauce to completely cover. Cover and cook on low for 8–10 hours or until chicken is thoroughly cooked.
3. In small bowl, combine cornstarch and water; stir until smooth. Add to slow cooker and stir. Cook on high for 15–20 minutes longer until sauce is thickened.

Nutrition Info:

- Per Serving: Calories: 236.53; Fat: 9.30 g ;Saturated fat:1.79 g;Sodium: 277.24 mg

Turkey Breast With Dried Fruit

Servings: 6

Cooking Time: X

Ingredients:

- 1½ pounds bone-in turkey breast
- 1/8 teaspoon salt
- 1/8 teaspoon pepper
- 1 tablespoon flour
- 1 tablespoon olive oil
- 1 tablespoon butter or plant sterol margarine
- ½ cup chopped prunes
- ½ cup chopped dried apricots
- 2 Granny Smith apples, peeled and chopped
- 1 cup Low-Sodium Chicken Broth
- ¼ cup Madeira wine

Directions:

1. Sprinkle turkey with salt, pepper, and flour. In large saucepan, heat olive oil and butter over medium heat. Add turkey and cook until browned, about 5 minutes. Turn turkey.
2. Add all fruit to saucepan along with broth and wine. Cover and bring to a simmer. Reduce heat to medium low and simmer for 55–65 minutes or until turkey is thoroughly cooked. Serve turkey with fruit and sauce.

Nutrition Info:

- Per Serving: Calories: 293.15; Fat: 6.01 g ;Saturated fat: 1.94 g ;Sodium: 127.28 mg

Turkey Tacos Verde

Servings: 4

Cooking Time: 13 Minutes

Ingredients:

- 1 teaspoon olive oil
- 1 pound 99% lean ground white turkey
- 1 onion, chopped
- 3 cloves garlic, minced
- 10 tomatillos, husk removed, rinsed and chopped
- 2 jalapeño peppers, seeded and minced
- ½ cup low-sodium salsa verde
- 8 corn tortillas, warmed
- ½ cup low-fat plain Greek yogurt
- 2 tablespoons chopped fresh cilantro
- 2 scallions, minced
- 2 cups mixed salad greens

Directions:

1. In a large nonstick skillet, heat the olive oil over medium heat.
2. Add the ground turkey, onion, and garlic and stir to break up the meat.
3. Sauté the mixture until the turkey is cooked through, about 5 to 6 minutes.
4. Add the tomatillos and jalapeño peppers and stir for 3 to 4 minutes. Then add the salsa verde and stir.
5. Meanwhile, combine the yogurt, cilantro, and scallions in a small bowl
6. Assemble the tacos starting with the tortillas, turkey mixture, yogurt mixture, and top with the salad greens. Serve immediately.

Nutrition Info:

- Per Serving: Calories:338 ; Fat : 6 g ;Saturated fat: 1 g ;Sodium: 295 mg

Chicken Poached In Tomato Sauce

Servings: 4

Cooking Time: X

Ingredients:

- 1 cup brown rice
- 2 cups water
- 2 tablespoons olive oil
- 1 onion, chopped
- 3 cloves garlic, minced
- 2 cups chopped plum tomatoes
- ½ teaspoon dried tarragon
- ¼ cup dry red wine
- 3 tablespoons no-salt tomato paste
- 1 cup Low-Sodium Chicken Broth
- 1/8 teaspoon salt
- 1/8 teaspoon pepper
- 3 (5-ounce) boneless, skinless chicken thighs, sliced

Directions:

1. In medium saucepan, combine rice and water and bring to a boil over high heat. Reduce heat to low, cover, and simmer for 30–40 minutes or until rice is tender.
2. Meanwhile, in large saucepan heat olive oil over medium heat. Add onion and garlic; cook and stir for 4 minutes until crisp-tender. Add tomatoes, tarragon, wine, tomato paste, chicken broth, salt, and pepper, and bring to a simmer, stirring frequently.
3. Add chicken and bring back to a simmer. Cover pan, reduce heat to low, and poach chicken for 15–20 minutes or until thoroughly cooked. Serve over hot cooked rice.

Nutrition Info:

- Per Serving: Calories: 285.33; Fat: 9.22g ;Saturated fat: 1.70 g;Sodium: 129.66 mg

Iron Packed Turkey

Servings: 2

Cooking Time: 30 Min

Ingredients:

- 2 (3 oz) turkey breasts, boneless and skinless
- Himalayan pink salt
- Ground black pepper
- 3 tsp avocado oil, divided
- 1 ½ cups spinach, roughly chopped
- 1 ½ cups kale, roughly chopped
- 1 ½ cups Swiss chard, roughly chopped
- 1 ½ cups collard greens, roughly chopped
- 1 tsp garlic crushed

Directions:

1. Preheat the oven to 400°F gas mark 6.
2. Season the turkey breasts with salt and pepper to taste.
3. Heat 1 tsp of avocado oil in a large cast-iron frying pan over medium-high heat.
4. Add the turkey breasts and cook for 5 minutes on each side until browned. Remove the turkey breasts and set them aside.
5. Add the remaining 2 tsp of avocado oil to the pan and fry the spinach, kale, Swiss chard, collard greens and garlic for 3 minutes until they are slightly wilted.
6. Season the mixed greens with salt and pepper to taste, place the turkey breasts on the greens.
7. Place the cast iron frying pan in the oven and bake for 15 minutes until the turkey breasts are cooked through.
8. Serve warm

Nutrition Info:

- Per Serving: Calories: 113 ; Fat: 2 g ;Saturated fat: 0 g ;Sodium: 128 mg

Cold Chicken With Cherry Tomato Sauce

Servings: 3

Cooking Time: X

Ingredients:

- 2 teaspoons fresh thyme leaves
- ½ cup Low-Sodium Chicken Broth
- 12 ounces boneless, skinless chicken breasts
- 1 tablespoon olive oil
- 3 cloves garlic, minced
- 2 cups cherry tomatoes
- ½ cup no-salt tomato juice
- ½ cup chopped fresh basil
- ¼ cup low-fat sour cream
- 1/8 teaspoon white pepper

Directions:

1. In large saucepan, combine thyme and chicken broth; bring to a simmer over medium heat. Add chicken and reduce heat to low. Cover and poach for 7–9 minutes or until chicken is thoroughly cooked.
2. Place chicken in a casserole dish just large enough to hold the chicken. Pour poaching liquid over, then cover and refrigerate for at least 8 hours.
3. When ready to eat, heat olive oil in large skillet. Add garlic; cook and stir for 1 minute. Then stir in cherry tomatoes; cook and stir until the tomatoes pop, about 4–6 minutes. Add tomato juice, basil, sour cream, and pepper; stir, and heat briefly.
4. Slice the chicken and fan out on serving plate. Top with tomato mixture and serve immediately.

Nutrition Info:

- Per Serving: Calories: 227.58; Fat: 8.63 g   ;Saturated fat: 2.57 g ;Sodium: 198.32 mg

Mini Turkey Meatloaves

Servings: 4

Cooking Time: 20 Minutes

Ingredients:

- ⅓ cup old-fashioned rolled oats
- 2 scallions, finely chopped
- 1 egg
- 3 tablespoons no-salt-added tomato paste, divided
- 2 teaspoons olive oil
- Pinch salt
- ⅛ teaspoon black pepper
- ½ teaspoon dried ground leaves
- 16 ounces 99% lean ground white turkey
- 2 tablespoons low-sodium mustard
- 1 tablespoon water

Directions:

1. Preheat the oven to 450°F. Line a baking sheet with aluminum foil.
2. In a large bowl, combine the oats, scallions, egg, 2 tablespoons of the tomato paste, olive oil, salt, pepper, and marjoram, and mix well.
3. Add the ground turkey, and mix gently with your hands until well combined.
4. Divide the mixture into fourths and shape into mini loaves. Place on the prepared baking sheet.
5. In a small bowl, combine the remaining 1 tablespoon tomato paste, the mustard, and water and mix well. Brush over the mini meatloaves.
6. Bake for 18 to 22 minutes or until the meatloaves register 165°F on a meat thermometer.

Nutrition Info:

- Per Serving: Calories: 205 ; Fat : 5 g ;Saturated fat: 1 g ;Sodium: 252 mg

Sesame-crusted Chicken

Servings: 4

Cooking Time: X

Ingredients:

- 2 tablespoons low-sodium soy sauce
- 2 cloves garlic, minced
- 1 tablespoon grated ginger root
- 1 tablespoon brown sugar
- 1 teaspoon sesame oil
- 4 (4-ounce) boneless, skinless chicken breasts
- ½ cup sesame seeds
- 3 tablespoons olive oil
- 1 tablespoon butter

Directions:

1. In large food storage heavy-duty plastic bag, combine soy sauce, garlic, ginger root, brown sugar, and sesame oil and mix well. Add chicken; seal bag, and squish to coat chicken with marinade. Place in bowl and refrigerate for 8 hours.
2. When ready to eat, remove chicken from marinade; discard marinade. Dip chicken in sesame seeds to coat on all sides.
3. Heat olive oil and butter in large skillet over medium heat. Add chicken and cook for 5 minutes. Carefully turn chicken and cook for 3–6 minutes on second side or until chicken is thoroughly cooked and sesame seeds are toasted. Serve immediately.

Nutrition Info:

- Per Serving: Calories: 363.65; Fat: 20.83 g ;Saturated fat:4.15 g;Sodium: 250.28 mg

Tomatoes With Chicken Mousse

Servings: 4

Cooking Time: X

Ingredients:

- 1 cup diced cooked chicken
- ¼ cup minced red onion
- 1 tablespoon chopped fresh chives
- 1 tablespoon fresh rosemary, minced
- 1/3 cup low-fat yogurt
- ¼ cup low-fat mayonnaise
- 1 tablespoon lime juice
- ½ cup chopped celery
- 4 large ripe tomatoes

Directions:

1. In blender or food processor, combine all ingredients except celery and tomatoes. Blend or process until smooth. Stir in celery.
2. Cut the tops off the tomatoes and scoop out the insides, leaving a " shell. Turn upside down on paper towels and let drain for 10 minutes.
3. Fill tomatoes with the chicken mixture and top each with the tomato top. Cover and chill for 2–3 hours before serving.

Nutrition Info:

- Per Serving: Calories:169.29; Fat: 7.01 g ;Saturated fat:1.41 g ;Sodium: 167.31 mg

Chicken Pesto

Servings: 6

Cooking Time: X

Ingredients:

- 1 cup packed fresh basil leaves
- ¼ cup toasted chopped hazelnuts
- 2 cloves garlic, chopped
- 2 tablespoons olive oil
- 1 tablespoons water
- ¼ cup grated Parmesan cheese
- ½ cup Low-Sodium Chicken Broth
- 12 ounces boneless, skinless chicken breasts
- 1 (12-ounce) package angel hair pasta

Directions:

1. Bring a large pot of salted water to a boil. In blender or food processor, combine basil, hazelnuts, and garlic. Blend or process until very finely chopped. Add olive oil and water; blend until a paste forms. Then blend in Parmesan cheese; set aside.
2. In large skillet, bring chicken broth to a simmer over medium heat. Cut chicken into strips and add to broth. Cook for 4 minutes, then add the pasta to the boiling water.
3. Cook pasta for 3–4 minutes according to package directions, until al dente. Drain and add to chicken mixture; cook and stir for 1 minute until chicken is thoroughly cooked. Add basil mixture, remove from heat, and stir until a sauce forms. Serve immediately.

Nutrition Info:

- Per Serving: Calories: 373.68; Fat: 11.06 g ;Saturated fat: 2.01 g ;Sodium: 108.92 mg

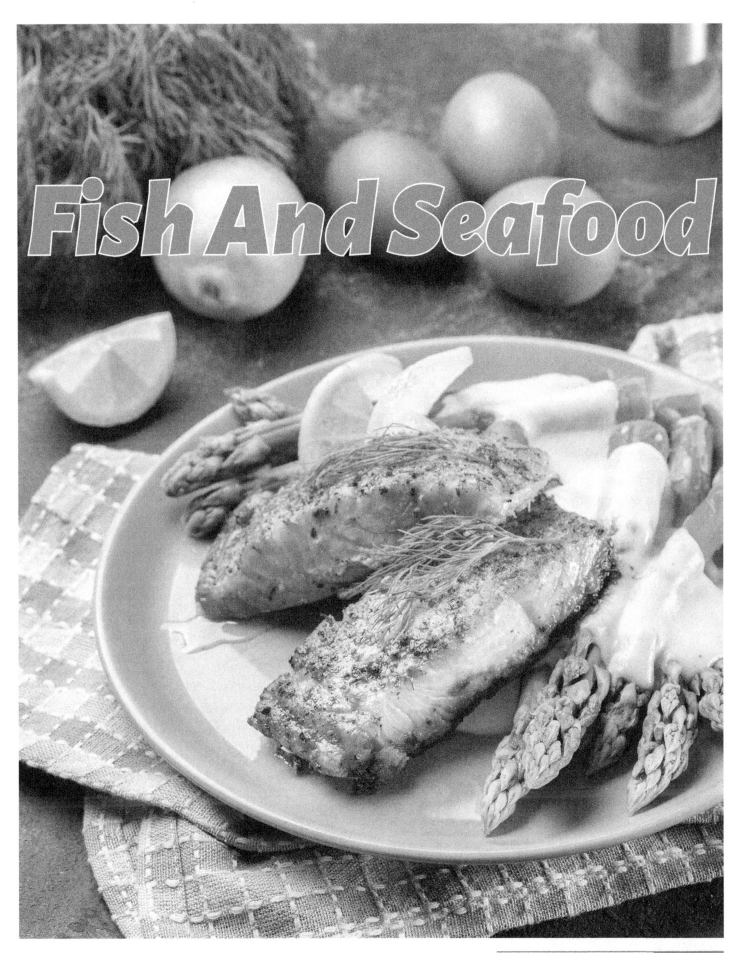

Fish And Seafood

Fish And Seafood

Salmon Vegetable Stir-fry

Servings: 4

Cooking Time: X

Ingredients:

- 2 tablespoons rice vinegar
- 1 tablespoon sugar
- 1 tablespoon grated ginger root
- 1 tablespoon cornstarch
- 2 tablespoons hoisin sauce
- 1/8 teaspoon white pepper
- 2 tablespoons peanut oil
- 1 onion, sliced
- ½ pound sugar-snap peas
- 3 carrots, sliced
- 1 red bell pepper, sliced
- ¼ pound salmon fillet

Directions:

1. In small bowl, combine rice vinegar, sugar, ginger root, cornstarch, hoi-sin sauce, and pepper. Mix well and set aside.
2. In large skillet or wok, heat peanut oil over high heat. Add onion, peas, and carrots. Stir-fry for 3–4 minutes or until vegetables begin to soften. Add red bell pepper.
3. Immediately place salmon fillet on top of vegetables. Reduce heat to medium, cover skillet or wok and cook for 4–5 minutes or until salmon flakes when tested with fork.
4. Stir the vinegar mixture and add to skillet or wok. Turn heat to medium-high and stir-fry to break up the salmon for 2–3 minutes until the sauce bubbles and thickens. Serve immediately over hot cooked rice.

Nutrition Info:

- Per Serving: Calories: 371.71; Fat:11.73 g ;Saturated fat: 3.24 g ;Sodium: 237.60 mg

Seared Scallops With Fruit

Servings: 3–4

Cooking Time: X

Ingredients:

- 1 pound sea scallops Pinch salt
- 1/8 teaspoon white pepper
- 1 tablespoon olive oil
- 1 tablespoon butter or margarine
- ¼ cup dry white wine
- 2 peaches, sliced
- 1 cup blueberries
- 1 tablespoon lime juice

Directions:

1. Rinse scallops and pat dry. Sprinkle with salt and pepper and set aside.
2. In large skillet, heat olive oil and butter over medium-high heat. Add the scallops and don't move them for 3 minutes. Carefully check to see if the scallops are deep golden brown. If they are, turn and cook for 1–2 minutes on the second side.
3. Remove scallops to serving plate. Add peaches to skillet and brown quickly on one side, about 2 minutes. Turn peaches and add wine to skillet; bring to a boil. Remove from heat and add blueberries. Pour over scallops, sprinkle with lime juice, and serve immediately.

Nutrition Info:

- Per Serving: Calories: 207.89; Fat: 7.36 g ;Saturated fat:2.40 g ;Sodium: 242.16 mg

Orange Thyme Red Snapper

Servings: 4

Cooking Time: 10 Minutes

Ingredients:

- 1 medium orange
- 2 teaspoons olive oil
- 4 (6-ounce) fillets red snapper
- Pinch salt
- ⅛ teaspoon white pepper
- 2 teaspoons olive oil
- 2 scallions, chopped
- 1½ teaspoons fresh thyme leaves, or ½ teaspoon dried

Directions:

1. Rinse the orange and dry. Using a small grater or zester, remove 1 teaspoon zest from the orange and set aside. Cut the orange in half, squeeze in a small bowl, and reserve the juice.
2. Add the olive oil to a large nonstick skillet and place over medium heat. Meanwhile, sprinkle the fish with the salt and white pepper.
3. Add the fish to the skillet, skin-side down, if the skin is attached. Cook 3 minutes on one side, briefly pressing on the fish with a spatula to prevent curling (or slit the fillet to prevent curling). Turn the fish and cook for 2 to 3 minutes on the second side, until the fish flakes when tested with a fork.
4. Transfer the fish to a plate. Remove the skin, if present, and discard. Cover the fish with a foil tent to keep it warm.
5. Add the scallions and the thyme to the skillet; cook and stir gently for 1 minute. Add the reserved orange juice and orange zest and simmer for 2 to 3 minutes or until the liquid is slightly reduced.
6. Pour the sauce over the fish and serve immediately.

Nutrition Info:

- Per Serving: Calories: 232 ; Fat: 7 g ;Saturated fat: 1 g;Sodium: 121 mg

Scallops On Skewers With Tomatoes

Servings: 4

Cooking Time: X

Ingredients:

- 1 pound sea scallops
- 12 cherry tomatoes
- 4 green onions, cut in half crosswise
- ½ cup chopped parsley
- 1 tablespoon fresh oregano leaves
- 3 tablespoons olive oil
- 2 tablespoons lemon juice
- 2 cloves garlic
- 1/8 teaspoon salt
- 1/8 teaspoon pepper

Directions:

1. Prepare and preheat broiler. Rinse scallops and pat dry. Thread on skewers along with cherry tomatoes and green onions.
2. In blender or food processor, combine remaining ingredients. Blend or process until smooth. Reserve ¼ cup of this sauce.
3. Brush remaining sauce onto the food on the skewers. Place on broiler pan. Broil 6″ from heat for 3–4 minutes per side, turning once during cooking time. Serve with remaining sauce.

Nutrition Info:

- Per Serving: Calories:202.03 ; Fat:11.11 g ;Saturated fat: 1.52 g ;Sodium:251.50 mg

Vietnamese Fish And Noodle Bowl

Servings: 3

Cooking Time: 15 Minutes

Ingredients:

- ¾ pound grouper fillets, cut into 1-inch pieces
- 1 tablespoon cornstarch
- ⅛ teaspoon cayenne pepper
- 2 teaspoons fish sauce
- 1 tablespoon rice wine vinegar
- 1 teaspoon sugar
- 2 tablespoons fresh lemon juice
- 1 teaspoon olive oil
- ¼ cup minced daikon radish
- 3 cloves garlic, minced
- 4 ounces whole-wheat spaghetti, broken in half
- 1½ cups low-sodium vegetable broth
- 2 tablespoons chopped peanuts
- 2 tablespoons minced fresh cilantro
- 2 tablespoons minced fresh basil

Directions:

1. In a medium bowl, toss the grouper with the cornstarch and cayenne pepper and set aside.
2. In a small bowl, combine the fish sauce, rice wine vinegar, sugar, and lemon juice, and stir to mix well.
3. In a large skillet, heat the olive oil over medium heat. Add the daikon and garlic and cook for 1 minute, stirring constantly.
4. Add the fish to the skillet; sauté for 2 to 3 minutes, stirring frequently, until the fish browns lightly.
5. Remove the fish mixture to a large bowl and set aside.
6. Add the spaghetti and vegetable broth to the skillet, and stir. Bring to a simmer over high heat and cook for 7 to 8 minutes or until the pasta is al dente.
7. Return the fish and radish mixture to the skillet along with the fish sauce mixture, peanuts, cilantro, and basil. Toss for 1 minute, then serve immediately in bowls.

Nutrition Info:

- Per Serving: Calories: 324 ; Fat: 6 g ;Saturated fat: 1 g;Sodium: 439 mg

Citrus Cod Bake

Servings: 2

Cooking Time: 25 Min

Ingredients:

- 2 tbsp. garlic, crushed
- 1 tbsp. olive oil
- 2 rosemary sprigs, stem removed and finely chopped
- 2 oregano sprigs, finely chopped
- 2 cod fillets, rinsed and patted dry
- ¼ tsp Himalayan pink salt
- ¼ tsp ground black pepper
- 1 lime, cut into 4 round slices
- ½ lemon, wedged

Directions:

1. Heat the oven to 450°F gas mark 8.
2. In a small-sized mixing bowl, add the garlic, olive oil, rosemary, and oregano, mix to combine.
3. Place the cod fillets on a baking sheet and season with salt and pepper.
4. Evenly coat both cod fillets with the garlic and herb mixture. Place 2 lime slices on each fillet. Bake for 18 to 25 minutes, or until the cod fillets are completely cooked.
5. Serve with a lemon wedge.

Nutrition Info:

- Per Serving: Calories: 218 ; Fat:3 g ;Saturated fat: 1 g ;Sodium: 430 mg

Citrus-blueberry Fish En Papillote

Servings: 4

Cooking Time: X

Ingredients:

- 1 tablespoon olive oil
- 1 onion, finely chopped
- 4 cloves garlic, minced
- 2 tablespoons lemon juice
- 2 tablespoons orange juice
- 1 teaspoon orange zest
- 4 (4-ounce) sole or mahi mahi fillets
- 1 cup blueberries
- 2 tablespoons blueberry jam

Directions:

1. Preheat oven to 400°F. Cut parchment paper into four large heart shapes measuring about 12″ × 18″. Fold hearts in half, open up, then set aside.
2. In small saucepan, heat olive oil over medium heat. Add onion and garlic; cook and stir for 4 minutes until crisp-tender. Remove from heat and stir in lemon and orange juice along with orange zest.
3. Place one fillet at the center of each parchment heart, next to the fold. Divide onion mixture among fillets. In small bowl, combine blueberries and blueberry jam and mix gently. Divide on top of onion mixture.
4. Fold one half of the parchment heart over the other. Crimp and fold the edges to seal. Place on cookie sheets. Bake for 18–23 minutes or until the bundles are puffed and the paper is browned.
5. Serve immediately, warning diners to be careful of the steam that will billow out when the packages are opened.

Nutrition Info:

- Per Serving: Calories:220.81 ; Fat:5.18 g ;Saturated fat:0.87 g ;Sodium:116.46 mg

Shrimp Stir-fry

Servings: 2

Cooking Time: 15 Min

Ingredients:

- 12 oz zucchini spirals
- 2 tsp low-sodium tamari sauce
- 2 tsp apple cider vinegar
- 1 tsp ginger, peeled and grated
- 1 tsp garlic, crushed
- 1 tsp organic honey
- 2 tsp sesame oil
- 6 oz shrimp, peeled and deveined
- 2 cups napa cabbage, shredded
- 1 medium green bell pepper, thinly sliced
- 1 spring onion, thinly sliced
- 1 tbsp. toasted sesame seeds, for garnish

Directions:

1. Cook the zucchini according to the package directions. Drain and run under cold water to stop the cooking process. Transfer the zucchini to a medium-sized mixing bowl and set aside.
2. In a small-sized mixing bowl, add the tamari sauce, apple cider vinegar, ginger, garlic, and honey, mix to combine, and set aside.
3. Warm the sesame oil in a medium-sized, heavy-bottom pan over medium-high heat. Add the shrimp and fry for 5 minutes until cooked through.
4. Add the napa cabbage, green bell pepper, and spring onion and fry for 4 minutes until the vegetables are tender. Add the tamari sauce mixture and the zucchini, toss to coat, heat for 1 minute.
5. Serve into bowls and top with sesame seeds.

Nutrition Info:

- Per Serving: Calories: 400 ; Fat: 8 g ;Saturated fat: 1 g ;Sodium: 347 mg

Cod Satay

Servings: 4

Cooking Time: 15 Minutes

Ingredients:

- 2 teaspoons olive oil, divided
- 1 small onion, diced
- 2 cloves garlic, minced
- ⅓ cup low-fat coconut milk
- 1 tomato, chopped
- 2 tablespoons low-fat peanut butter
- 1 tablespoon packed brown sugar
- ⅓ cup low-sodium vegetable broth
- 2 teaspoons low-sodium soy sauce
- ⅛ teaspoon ground ginger
- Pinch red pepper flakes
- 4 (6-ounce) cod fillets
- ⅛ teaspoon white pepper

Directions:

1. In a small saucepan, heat 1 teaspoon of the olive oil over medium heat.
2. Add the onion and garlic, and cook, stirring frequently for 3 minutes.
3. Add the coconut milk, tomato, peanut butter, brown sugar, broth, soy sauce, ginger, and red pepper flakes, and bring to a simmer, stirring with a whisk until the sauce combines. Simmer for 2 minutes, then remove the satay sauce from the heat and set aside.
4. Season the cod with the white pepper.
5. Heat a large nonstick skillet with the remaining 1 teaspoon olive oil, and add the cod fillets. Cook for 3 minutes, then turn and cook for 3 to 4 minutes more or until the fish flakes when tested with a fork.
6. Cover the fish with the satay sauce and serve immediately.

Nutrition Info:

- Per Serving: Calories: 255 ; Fat: 10 g ;Saturated fat: 5 g;Sodium: 222 mg

Halibut Parcels

Servings: 4

Cooking Time: 15 Min

Ingredients:

- Aluminum foil
- 4 cups kale, stems removed and shredded
- 2 cups button mushrooms, sliced
- 4 (4 oz) halibut fillets
- ½ tsp seafood seasoning
- ½ tsp fine sea salt
- ¼ tsp ground black pepper
- ¼ cup spring onion, chopped
- 2 tbsp. olive oil

Directions:

1. Heat the oven to 425°F gas mark 7.
2. Prepare the aluminum foil by tearing them into squares, big enough for the fillets and vegetables.
3. Place 1 cup of kale and ½ cup of mushroom onto each foil square.
4. Place the halibut fillet on top of each parcel. Season with seafood seasoning, salt and pepper.
5. Sprinkle the spring onion over this and drizzle with olive oil.
6. Fold the foil to seal in the halibut and vegetables.
7. Place on a baking sheet and bake for 15 minutes. Remove from the oven and carefully unfold the parcels.

Nutrition Info:

- Per Serving: Calories:155 ; Fat: 7 g ;Saturated fat: 1 g ;Sodium: 435 mg

Seafood Risotto

Servings: 6

Cooking Time: X

Ingredients:

- 2 cups water
- 2½ cups Low-Sodium Chicken Broth
- 2 tablespoons olive oil
- 1 onion, minced
- 3 cloves garlic, minced
- 1½ cups Arborio rice
- 1 cup chopped celery
- 1 tablespoon fresh dill weed
- ¼ cup dry white wine
- ½ pound sole fillets
- ¼ pound small raw shrimp
- ½ pound bay scallops
- ¼ cup grated Parmesan cheese
- 1 tablespoon butter

Directions:

1. In medium saucepan, combine water and broth and heat over low heat. Keep mixture on heat.
2. In large saucepan, heat olive oil over medium heat. Add onion and garlic; cook and stir until crisp-tender, about 3 minutes. Add rice; cook and stir for 3 minutes.
3. Start adding broth mixture, a cup at a time, stirring frequently, adding liquid when previous addition is absorbed. When only 1 cup of broth remains to be added, stir in celery, dill, wine, fish fillets, shrimp, and scallops to rice mixture. Add last cup of broth.
4. Cook, stirring constantly, for 5–7 minutes or until fish is cooked and rice is tender and creamy. Stir in Parmesan and butter, stir, and serve.

Nutrition Info:

- Per Serving: Calories:397.22 ; Fat:11.11 g ;Saturated fat:3.20 g ;Sodium:354.58 mg

Salmon With Farro Pilaf

Servings: 4

Cooking Time: 25 Minutes

Ingredients:

- ½ cup farro
- 1¼ cups low-sodium vegetable broth
- 4 (4-ounce) salmon fillets
- Pinch salt
- ½ teaspoon dried marjoram leaves
- ⅛ teaspoon white pepper
- ¼ cup dried cherries
- ¼ cup dried currants
- 1 cup fresh baby spinach leaves
- 1 tablespoon orange juice

Directions:

1. Preheat the oven to 400°F. Line a baking sheet with parchment paper and set aside.
2. In a medium saucepan over medium heat, combine the farro and the vegetable broth and bring to a simmer. Reduce the heat to low and simmer, partially covered, for 25 minutes, or until the farro is tender.
3. Meanwhile, sprinkle the salmon with the salt, marjoram, and white pepper and place on the prepared baking sheet.
4. When the farro has cooked for 10 minutes, bake the salmon in the oven for 12 to 15 minutes, or until the salmon flakes when tested with a fork. Remove and cover to keep warm.
5. When the farro is tender, add the cherries, currants, spinach, and orange juice; stir and cover. Let stand off the heat for 2 to 3 minutes.
6. Plate the salmon and serve with the farro pilaf.

Nutrition Info:

- Per Serving: Calories: 304 ; Fat: 8 g ;Saturated fat: 2 g;Sodium: 139 mg

Sesame-pepper Salmon Kabobs

Servings: 4

Cooking Time: X

Ingredients:

- 1 pound salmon steak
- 2 tablespoons olive oil, divided
- ¼ cup sesame seeds
- 1 teaspoon pepper
- 1 red bell pepper
- 1 yellow bell pepper
- 1 red onion
- 8 cremini mushrooms
- 1/8 teaspoon salt

Directions:

1. Prepare and preheat grill. Cut salmon steak into 1″ pieces, discarding skin and bones. Brush salmon with half of the olive oil.
2. In small bowl, combine sesame seeds and pepper and mix. Press all sides of salmon cubes into the sesame seed mixture.
3. Slice bell peppers into 1″ slices and cut red onion into 8 wedges; trim mushroom stems and leave caps whole. Skewer coated salmon pieces, peppers, onion, and mushrooms on metal skewers. Brush vegetables with remaining olive oil and sprinkle with salt.
4. Grill 6″ from medium coals, turning once during cooking time, until the sesame seeds are very brown and toasted and fish is just done, about 6–8 minutes. Serve immediately.

Nutrition Info:

- Per Serving: Calories:319.33 ; Fat:20.26 g ;Saturated fat: 3.67 g ;Sodium:141.88 mg

Roasted Shrimp And Veggies

Servings: 4

Cooking Time: 20 Minutes

Ingredients:

- 1 cup sliced cremini mushrooms
- 2 medium chopped Yukon Gold potatoes, rinsed, unpeeled
- 2 cups broccoli florets
- 3 cloves garlic, sliced
- 1 cup sliced fresh green beans
- 1 cup cauliflower florets
- 2 tablespoons fresh lemon juice
- 2 tablespoons low-sodium vegetable broth
- 1 teaspoon olive oil
- 1 teaspoon dried thyme
- ½ teaspoon dried oregano
- Pinch salt
- ⅛ teaspoon black pepper
- ½ pound medium shrimp, peeled and deveined

Directions:

1. Preheat the oven to 400°F.
2. In a large baking pan, combine the mushrooms, potatoes, broccoli, garlic, green beans, and cauliflower, and toss to coat.
3. In a small bowl, combine the lemon juice, broth, olive oil, thyme, oregano, salt, and pepper and mix well. Drizzle over the vegetables
4. Roast for 15 minutes, then stir.
5. Add the shrimp and distribute evenly.
6. Roast for another 5 minutes or until the shrimp curl and turn pink. Serve immediately.

Nutrition Info:

- Per Serving: Calories:192 ; Fat: 3 g ;Saturated fat: 0 g;Sodium: 116 mg

Steamed Sole Rolls With Greens

Servings: 4

Cooking Time: 10 Minutes

Ingredients:

- 4 (6-ounce) sole fillets
- 2 teaspoons grated peeled fresh ginger root
- 2 cloves garlic, minced
- 2 teaspoons low-sodium soy sauce
- 1 tablespoon rice wine vinegar
- 1 teaspoon toasted sesame oil
- 2 cups fresh torn spinach leaves
- 1 cup fresh stemmed torn kale
- 1 cup sliced mushrooms
- 2 teaspoons toasted sesame seeds

Directions:

1. Cut the sole fillets in half lengthwise. Sprinkle each piece with some of the ginger root and garlic. Roll up the fillets, ginger root side in. Fasten with a toothpick and set aside.
2. In a small bowl, combine the soy sauce, vinegar, and toasted sesame oil.
3. Bring water to a boil over medium heat in a large shallow saucepan that will hold your steamer.
4. Arrange the spinach leaves and kale in the bottom of the steamer. Add the rolled sole fillets. Add the mushrooms, and sprinkle everything with the soy sauce mixture.
5. Cover and steam for 7 to 11 minutes or until the fish is cooked and flakes when tested with a fork. Remove the toothpicks.
6. To serve, sprinkle with the sesame seeds and serve the fish on top of the wilted greens and mushrooms.

Nutrition Info:

- Per Serving: Calories: 263 ; Fat: 8 g ;Saturated fat: 2 g;Sodium: 247 mg

Shrimp And Pineapple Lettuce Wraps

Servings: 4

Cooking Time: 12 Minutes

Ingredients:

- 2 teaspoons olive oil
- 2 jalapeño peppers, seeded and minced
- 6 scallions, chopped
- 2 yellow bell peppers, seeded and chopped
- 8 ounces small shrimp, peeled and deveined
- 2 cups canned pineapple chunks, drained, reserving juice
- 2 tablespoons fresh lime juice
- 1 avocado, peeled, and cubed
- 1 large carrot, coarsely grated
- 8 romaine or Boston lettuce leaves, rinsed and dried

Directions:

1. In a medium saucepan, heat the olive oil over medium heat.
2. Add the jalapeño pepper and scallions and cook for 2 minutes, stirring constantly.
3. Add the bell pepper, and cook for 2 minutes.
4. Add the shrimp, and cook for 1 minute, stirring constantly.
5. Add the pineapple, 2 tablespoons of the reserved pineapple juice, and lime juice, and bring to a simmer. Simmer for 1 minute longer or until the shrimp curl and turn pink. Let the mixture cool for 5 minutes.
6. Serve the shrimp mixture with the cubed avocado and grated carrot, wrapped in the lettuce leaves.

Nutrition Info:

- Per Serving: Calories: 241 ; Fat: 9 g ;Saturated fat: 2 g;Sodium: 109 mg

Salmon With Mustard And Orange

Servings: 4

Cooking Time: X

Ingredients:

- 4 (5-ounce) salmon fillets
- 1 tablespoon olive oil
- 2 tablespoons Dijon mustard
- 1 tablespoon flour
- 1 teaspoon orange zest
- 2 tablespoons orange juice Pinch salt
- 1/8 teaspoon white pepper

Directions:

1. Preheat broiler. Place fillets on a broiler pan. In small bowl, combine remaining ingredients and mix well. Spread over salmon.
2. Broil fish 6″ from heat for 7–10 minutes or until fish flakes when tested with fork and topping bubbles and begins to brown. Serve immediately.

Nutrition Info:

- Per Serving: Calories: 277.64; Fat:14.02 g ;Saturated fat:2.09 g ;Sodium:197.84 mg

Cajun-rubbed Fish

Servings: 4

Cooking Time: X

Ingredients:

- ½ teaspoon black pepper
- ¼ teaspoon cayenne pepper
- ½ teaspoon lemon zest
- ½ teaspoon dried dill weed
- 1/8 teaspoon salt
- 1 tablespoon brown sugar
- 4 (5-ounce) swordfish steaks

Directions:

1. Prepare and preheat grill. In small bowl, combine pepper, cayenne pepper, lemon zest, dill weed, salt, and

brown sugar and mix well. Sprinkle onto both sides of the swordfish steaks and rub in. Set aside for 30 minutes.
2. Brush grill with oil. Add swordfish; cook without moving for 4 minutes. Then carefully turn steaks and cook for 2–4 minutes on second side until fish just flakes when tested with fork. Serve immediately.

Nutrition Info:

- Per Serving: Calories: 233.57 ; Fat:7.31 g ;Saturated fat: 2.00 g ;Sodium: 237.08 mg

Fried Mahi-mahi

Servings: 4

Cooking Time: 20 Min

Ingredients:

- 1 lb. mahi-mahi fillets
- ½ tsp fine sea salt
- ¼ tsp ground black pepper
- 1 tbsp. olive oil
- 1 medium green bell pepper, cored and chopped
- 1 small brown onion, chopped
- 2 cups grape tomatoes
- ¼ cup black olives, pitted and chopped

Directions:

1. Season the mahi-mahi fillets with salt and pepper.
2. Heat the olive oil in a large nonstick frying pan over medium-high heat.
3. Add the green bell pepper and onion. Cook for 3 to 5 minutes, until softened.
4. Add the grape tomatoes and black olives. Mix for 1 to 2 minutes, until the tomatoes have softened.
5. Place the mahi-mahi fillets on top of the vegetables and cover with a lid. Cook for 5 to 10 minutes, or until the fish flakes with a fork. Remove from the heat and serve.

Nutrition Info:

- Per Serving: Calories: 151 ; Fat: 5 g ;Saturated fat: 1 g ;Sodium: 603 mg

Cod And Potatoes

Servings: 4

Cooking Time: X

Ingredients:

- 3 Yukon Gold potatoes
- ¼ cup olive oil
- 1/8 teaspoon white pepper
- 1½ teaspoons dried herbs de Provence, divided
- 4 (4-ounce) cod steaks
- 1 tablespoon butter or margarine
- 2 tablespoons lemon juice

Directions:

1. Preheat oven to 350°F. Spray a 9″ glass baking dish with nonstick cooking spray. Thinly slice the potatoes. Layer in the baking dish, drizzling each layer with a tablespoon of olive oil, a sprinkle of pepper, and some of the herbs de Provence.
2. Bake for 35–45 minutes or until potatoes are browned on top and tender when pierced with a fork. Arrange cod steaks on top of potatoes. Dot with butter and sprinkle with lemon juice and remaining herbs de Provence.
3. Bake for 15–25 minutes longer or until fish flakes when tested with fork.

Nutrition Info:

- Per Serving: Calories: 362.62 ; Fat:17.28 g ;Saturated fat: 3.88 g ;Sodium: 91.56 mg

Tilapia Mint Wraps

Servings: 2

Cooking Time: 15 Min

Ingredients:

- Aluminum foil
- 2 (4 oz) tilapia fillets
- 1 tsp olive oil, divided
- ½ tsp seasoning rub blend, divided
- 4 iceberg lettuce leaves, divided
- 4 tbsp. mint sauce
- 1 tbsp. parsley, finely chopped

Directions:

1. Heat the oven to 425°F gas mark 7. Line a baking sheet with aluminum foil.
2. Place the tilapia fillets on the prepared baking sheet and season with olive oil and the seasoning rub blend.
3. Bake in the oven for 12 to 15 minutes, until the fish is fully cooked and flaky.
4. In the meantime, place the lettuce leaves onto serving plates.
5. When the fish is done, add 1 tbsp. of the mint sauce, ½ tbsp. parsley, and 2 oz of tilapia fillets per lettuce leaf and wrap tightly. Place two wraps on each plate and serve at room temperature.

Nutrition Info:

- Per Serving: Calories: 182 ; Fat: 6 g ;Saturated fat: 1 g ;Sodium: 114mg

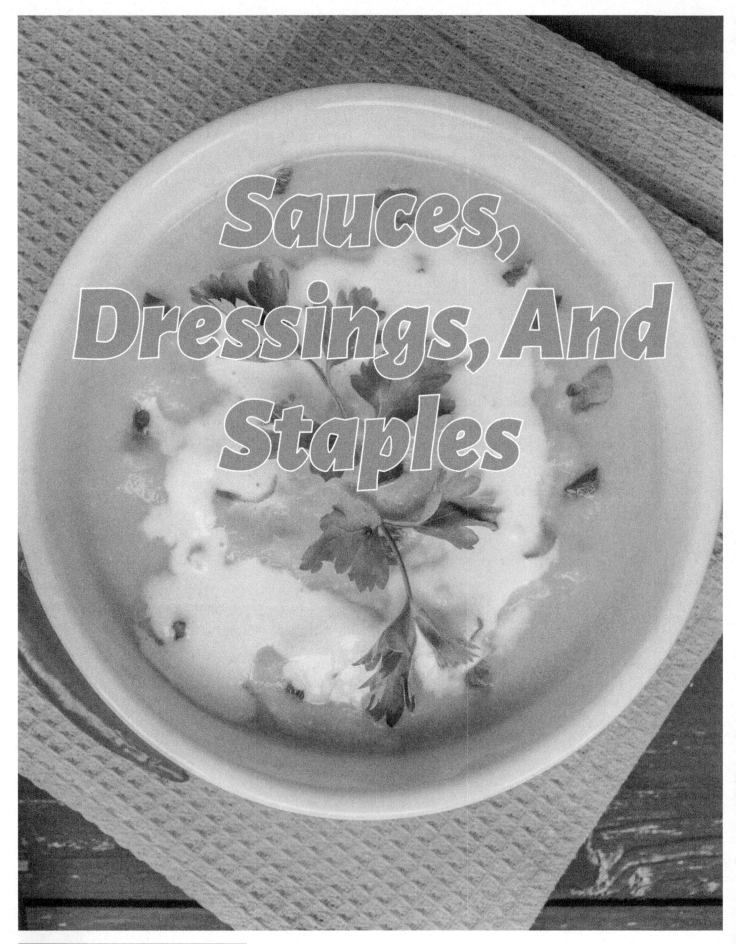

Sauces, Dressings, And Staples

Sauces, Dressings, And Staples

Mango, Peach, And Tomato Pico De Gallo

Servings: 4

Cooking Time: 15 Minutes

Ingredients:

- 1 mango, peeled and cubed (see Ingredient Tip)
- 1 peach, peeled and chopped (see Ingredient Tip)
- 1 beefsteak tomato, cored and chopped
- 1 cup yellow or red cherry tomatoes, chopped
- 2 scallions, chopped
- 1 jalapeño pepper, seeded and minced
- 2 tablespoons fresh lemon juice
- 1 teaspoon fresh grated lemon zest
- Pinch salt
- ⅛ teaspoon red pepper flakes

Directions:

1. In a medium bowl, combine the mango, peach, tomato, scallions, jalapeño pepper, lemon juice, lemon zest, salt, and red pepper flakes, and mix well.
2. Serve immediately or store in an airtight glass container in the refrigerator for up to 2 days.

Nutrition Info:

- Per Serving: Calories: 80 ; Fat: 1 g ;Saturated fat: 0 g ;Sodium: 48 mg

Sweet Salad Dressing

Servings: 5

Cooking Time: X

Ingredients:

- ¼ cup low-sodium Worcestershire sauce (or ¼ cup Worcestershire sauce)
- 2 tablespoons minced garlic
- 1½ tablespoons honey
- 2 teaspoons onion powder
- ½ teaspoon freshly ground black pepper

Directions:

1. In a small bowl, mix the Worcestershire sauce, garlic, honey, onion powder, and pepper until well blended. Use immediately.

Nutrition Info:

- Per Serving: Calories: 39 ; Fat: 0g ;Saturated fat: 0g ;Sodium: 136mg

Oregano-thyme Sauce

Servings: 5

Cooking Time: X

Ingredients:

- 2 tablespoons balsamic vinegar
- 1 tablespoon dried oregano
- 1 tablespoon dried thyme
- 1 tablespoon minced garlic
- ½ teaspoon salt

Directions:

1. In a small bowl, mix the vinegar, oregano, thyme, garlic, and salt until well blended. Use immediately

Nutrition Info:

- Per Serving: Calories: 10 ; Fat: 0 g ;Saturated fat: 0 g ;Sodium: 235 mg

Classic Italian Tomato Sauce

Servings: 4

Cooking Time: 20 Minutes

Ingredients:

- 2 teaspoons olive oil
- 1 onion, chopped
- 3 cloves garlic, minced
- 1½ pounds plum (Roma) tomatoes, chopped
- 2 tablespoons no-salt-added tomato paste
- 2 tablespoons finely grated carrot
- 1 teaspoon dried basil leaves
- ½ teaspoon dried oregano
- ⅛ teaspoon white pepper
- Pinch salt
- Pinch sugar
- 2 tablespoons fresh basil leaves, chopped

Directions:

1. In a large saucepan, heat the olive oil over medium heat.
2. Add the onion and garlic, and cook and stir for 3 minutes or until the onions are translucent.
3. Add the tomatoes, tomato paste, carrot, basil, oregano, white pepper, salt, and sugar, and stir and bring to a simmer.
4. Simmer for 15 to 18 minutes, stirring frequently, or until the sauce thickens slightly.
5. Stir in the fresh basil and serve.

Nutrition Info:

- Per Serving: Calories: 73 ; Fat: 3 g ;Saturated fat: 0 g ;Sodium: 19 mg

Spinach And Walnut Pesto

Servings: 5

Cooking Time: X

Ingredients:

- 2 cups spinach
- ½ cup chopped walnuts
- ½ cup olive oil
- 2 tablespoons minced garlic
- ½ teaspoon salt

Directions:

1. In a blender, place the spinach, walnuts, olive oil, garlic, and salt and blend until smooth. Use immediately.

Nutrition Info:

- Per Serving: Calories: 275 ; Fat: 29 g ;Saturated fat: 4g ;Sodium: 243 mg

Lemon-cilantro Vinaigrette

Servings: ⅓

Cooking Time: X

Ingredients:

- 2 tablespoons freshly squeezed lemon juice
- 2 tablespoons chopped fresh cilantro
- 2 tablespoons chopped jalapeño pepper
- 1 teaspoon honey
- ½ teaspoon minced garlic
- Pinch sea salt
- Pinch freshly ground black pepper
- Pinch cayenne pepper
- ¼ cup olive oil

Directions:

1. In a blender, add the lemon juice, cilantro, jalapeños, honey, garlic, salt, pepper, and cayenne and pulse until very smooth.
2. Turn the blender on and pour in the olive oil in a thin stream.

Nutrition Info:

- Per Serving: Calories: 117 ; Fat: 13 g ;Saturated fat: 2 g ;Sodium: 60 mg

Avocado Dressing

Servings: 8

Cooking Time: 15 Minutes

Ingredients:

- 1 avocado, peeled and cubed
- ⅔ cup plain nonfat Greek yogurt
- ¼ cup buttermilk
- 2 tablespoons fresh lemon juice
- 1 tablespoon honey
- Pinch salt
- 2 tablespoons chopped fresh chives
- ½ cup chopped cherry tomatoes

Directions:

1. In a blender or food processor, combine the avocado, yogurt, buttermilk, lemon juice, honey, salt, and chives, and blend or process until smooth. Stir in the tomatoes.
2. You may need to add more buttermilk or lemon juice to achieve a pourable consistency.
3. This dressing can be stored by putting it into a small dish, then pouring about 2 teaspoons lemon juice on top. Cover the dressing by pressing plastic wrap directly onto the surface. Refrigerate for up to 1 day.

Nutrition Info:

- Per Serving: Calories:55 ; Fat: 3g ;Saturated fat: 1g ;Sodium: 30mg

Sun-dried Tomato And Kalamata Olive Tapenade

Servings: 1¼

Cooking Time: X

Ingredients:

- ½ cup chopped sun-dried tomatoes

- ½ cup packed fresh basil leaves
- ¼ cup sliced Kalamata olives
- ¼ cup Parmesan cheese
- 2 garlic cloves
- 1 tablespoon olive oil
- Sea salt
- Freshly ground black pepper

Directions:

1. In a food processor or blender, place the sun-dried tomatoes, basil, olives, Parmesan cheese, garlic, and olive oil and pulse until smooth.
2. Season with salt and pepper.

Nutrition Info:

- Per Serving: Calories: 57 ; Fat: 3 g ;Saturated fat: 1 g ;Sodium: 207 mg

Simple Dijon And Honey Vinaigrette

Servings: ⅓

Cooking Time: X

Ingredients:

- 3 tablespoons olive oil
- 1½ tablespoons apple cider vinegar
- 1 tablespoon honey
- 2 teaspoons Dijon mustard
- Freshly ground black pepper

Directions:

1. In a small bowl, whisk together the oil, vinegar, honey, and mustard until emulsified.
2. Season with pepper and serve.

Nutrition Info:

- Per Serving: Calories: 145 ; Fat: 14 g ;Saturated fat: 2 g ;Sodium: 38 mg

Spicy Peanut Sauce

Servings: 8

Cooking Time: 15 Minutes

Ingredients:

- ½ cup powdered peanut butter (see Ingredient Tip)
- 2 tablespoons reduced-fat peanut butter
- ⅓ cup plain nonfat Greek yogurt
- 2 tablespoons fresh lime juice
- 2 teaspoons low-sodium soy sauce
- 1 scallion, chopped
- 1 clove garlic, minced
- 1 jalapeño pepper, seeded and minced
- ⅛ teaspoon red pepper flakes

Directions:

1. In a blender or food processor, combine powdered peanut butter, reduced-fat peanut butter, yogurt, lime juice, soy sauce, scallion, garlic, jalapeño pepper, and red pepper flakes, and blend or process until smooth.
2. Serve immediately or store in an airtight glass container and refrigerate for up to 3 days. You can thin this sauce with more lime juice if necessary.

Nutrition Info:

- Per Serving: Calories: 60 ; Fat: 3 g ;Saturated fat: 0 g ;Sodium: 88 mg

Chimichurri Sauce

Servings: 8

Cooking Time: 15 Minutes

Ingredients:

- 1 shallot, chopped
- 1 garlic clove, chopped
- ½ cup fresh flat-leaf parsley
- ½ cup fresh cilantro leaves
- 3 tablespoons fresh basil leaves
- 2 tablespoons fresh lemon juice
- 2 tablespoons low-sodium vegetable broth
- Pinch salt
- ⅛ teaspoon red pepper flakes

Directions:

1. In a blender or food processor, add the shallot, garlic, parsley, cilantro, basil, lemon juice, vegetable broth, salt, and red pepper flakes, and process until the herbs are in tiny pieces and the mixture is well-combined.
2. Serve immediately or store in an airtight glass container in the refrigerator up to 2 days. Stir the sauce before serving.

Nutrition Info:

- Per Serving: Calories: 5 ; Fat: 0 g ;Saturated fat: 0 g ;Sodium: 3 mg

Tofu-horseradish Sauce

Servings: X

Cooking Time: X

Ingredients:

- ¼ cup silken tofu
- 1 tablespoon prepared horscradish
- 1 tablespoon minced scallion, white part only
- 1 tablespoon chopped fresh parsley
- ½ teaspoon minced garlic
- Sea salt
- Freshly ground black pepper

Directions:

1. In a small bowl, stir together the tofu, horseradish, scallions, parsley, and garlic until well mixed.
2. Season with salt and pepper.
3. Serve immediately.

Nutrition Info:

- Per Serving: Calories: 20 ; Fat: 0 g ;Saturated fat: 0 g ;Sodium: 50 mg

Cheesy Spinach Dip

Servings: 1½

Cooking Time: 25 Minutes

Ingredients:

- 1 cup thawed chopped frozen spinach
- ½ cup fat-free cottage cheese
- 2 tablespoons chopped sweet onion
- ¼ cup grated Parmesan cheese
- 1 teaspoon minced garlic
- Sea salt
- Freshly ground black pepper

Directions:

1. In a medium bowl, stir together the spinach, cottage cheese, onion, Parmesan cheese, and garlic until well combined.
2. Season with salt and pepper.
3. Place the dip, covered, in the refrigerator until you are ready to serve it.
4. Serve with vegetables or pita bread.

Nutrition Info:

- Per Serving: Calories: 79 ; Fat: 2 g ;Saturated fat: 1 g ;Sodium: 213 mg

Zesty Citrus Kefir Dressing

Servings: 8

Cooking Time: 15 Minutes

Ingredients:

- ⅔ cup kefir
- 2 tablespoons honey
- 2 tablespoons low-sodium yellow mustard
- 2 tablespoons fresh lemon juice
- ½ teaspoon fresh lemon zest
- 1 tablespoon fresh orange juice
- ½ teaspoon fresh orange zest
- 1 teaspoon olive oil
- Pinch salt

Directions:

1. In a blender or food processor, combine the kefir, honey, mustard, lemon juice and zest, orange juice and zest, olive oil, and salt. Blend or process until smooth.
2. You can serve this dressing immediately, or store it in an airtight container in the refrigerator for up to 3 days.

Nutrition Info:

- Per Serving: Calories: 37 ; Fat: 1 g ;Saturated fat: 0 g ;Sodium: 43 mg

Mustard Berry Vinaigrette

Servings: 8

Cooking Time: 10 Minutes

Ingredients:

- 3 tablespoons low-sodium yellow mustard
- ½ cup fresh raspberries
- ½ cup sliced fresh strawberries
- 2 tablespoons raspberry vinegar
- 2 teaspoons agave nectar
- Pinch salt

Directions:

1. In a blender or food processor, combine the mustard, raspberries, strawberries, raspberry vinegar, agave nectar, and salt, and blend or process until smooth. You can also combine the ingredients in a bowl and mash them with the back of a fork.
2. Store the vinaigrette in an airtight glass container in the refrigerator for up to 3 days.

Nutrition Info:

- Per Serving: Calories: 27 ; Fat: 1 g ;Saturated fat: 0 g ;Sodium: 65 mg

Honey-garlic Sauce

Servings: 5

Cooking Time: X

Ingredients:

- 2 tablespoons low-sodium soy sauce (or 1 tablespoon soy sauce)
- 1½ tablespoons honey
- 1 tablespoon minced garlic
- 2 teaspoons sesame oil
- 1 teaspoon freshly ground black pepper

Directions:

1. In a small bowl, mix the soy sauce, honey, garlic, sesame oil, and pepper together until well blended and use immediately.

Nutrition Info:

- Per Serving: Calories: 42 ; Fat: 2g ;Saturated fat: 0g ;Sodium: 205mg

Green Sauce

Servings: 4

Cooking Time: 15 Minutes

Ingredients:

- 1 cup watercress
- ½ cup frozen baby peas, thawed
- ¼ cup chopped fresh cilantro leaves
- 2 scallions, chopped
- 3 tablespoons silken tofu
- 2 tablespoons fresh lime juice
- 1 tablespoon green olive slices
- 1 teaspoon grated fresh lime zest
- Pinch salt
- Pinch white pepper

Directions:

1. In a food processor or blender, combine the watercress, peas, cilantro, scallions, tofu, lime juice, olives, lime zest, salt, and white pepper, and process or blend until smooth.
2. This sauce can be used immediately, or you can store it in an airtight glass container in the refrigerator up to four days.

Nutrition Info:

- Per Serving: Calories: 27 ; Fat: 1 g ;Saturated fat: 0 g ;Sodium: 65 mg

Buttermilk-herb Dressing

Servings: ¾

Cooking Time: X

Ingredients:

- ½ cup buttermilk
- ¼ cup silken tofu
- 2 tablespoons minced scallion, white part only
- 1 tablespoon chopped fresh parsley
- 1 tablespoon chopped fresh thyme
- 1 teaspoon chopped fresh dill
- Sea salt
- Freshly ground black pepper

Directions:

1. In a medium bowl, whisk together the buttermilk, tofu, scallions, parsley, thyme, and dill until well blended.
2. Season with salt and pepper.

Nutrition Info:

- Per Serving: Calories: 17 ; Fat: 0 g ;Saturated fat: 0 g ;Sodium: 35 mg

Tzatziki

Servings: 4

Cooking Time: X

Ingredients:

- 1¼ cups plain low-fat Greek yogurt
- 1 cucumber, peeled, seeded, and diced
- 2 tablespoons fresh lime juice
- ½ teaspoon grated fresh lime zest
- 2 cloves garlic, minced
- Pinch salt
- ⅛ teaspoon white pepper
- 1 tablespoon minced fresh dill
- 1 tablespoon minced fresh mint
- 2 teaspoons olive oil

Directions:

1. In a medium bowl, combine the yogurt, cucumber, lime juice, lime zest, garlic, salt, white pepper, dill, and mint.
2. Transfer the mixture to a serving bowl. Drizzle with the olive oil.
3. Serve immediately or store in an airtight glass container and refrigerate for up to 2 days

Nutrition Info:

- Per Serving: Calories: 100 ; Fat: 4 g ;Saturated fat: 1 g ;Sodium: 56 mg

Spicy Honey Sauce

Servings: 5

Cooking Time: X

Ingredients:

- 2 tablespoons vegetable oil
- 1½ tablespoons honey
- 1 tablespoon minced garlic
- 1 tablespoon chili powder
- ½ teaspoon salt

Directions:

1. In a small bowl, mix the vegetable oil, honey, garlic, chili powder, and salt until well blended. Use immediately.

Nutrition Info:

- Per Serving: Calories: 78 ; Fat: 6 g ;Saturated fat: 0 g ;Sodium: 279 mg

Smoky Barbecue Rub

Servings: ½

Cooking Time: X

Ingredients:

- 2 tablespoons smoked paprika
- 2 tablespoons brown sugar
- 1 tablespoon chili powder
- 1 tablespoon garlic powder
- 2 teaspoons onion powder
- 2 teaspoons celery salt
- 1 teaspoon ground cumin
- ½ teaspoon sea salt
- ½ teaspoon dried oregano

Directions:

1. In a small bowl, whisk together the paprika, sugar, chili powder, garlic powder, onion powder, celery salt, cumin, salt, and oregano until well blended.
2. Transfer to an airtight container to store.

Nutrition Info:

- Per Serving: Calories: 23 ; Fat: 1 g ;Saturated fat: 0 g ;Sodium: 113 mg

Desserts And Treats

Low Cholesterol
Cookbook

Desserts And Treats

Lite Creamy Cheesecake

Servings: 12

Cooking Time: X

Ingredients:

- 1½ cups crushed gingersnap crumbs
- 1/3 cup finely chopped walnuts
- 2 tablespoons butter or margarine, melted
- 2 tablespoons orange juice
- 1½ cups nonfat cottage cheese
- 1 cup sugar
- ¼ cup orange juice
- 2 tablespoons lemon juice
- 1 (8-ounce) package light cream cheese, softened 1 (3-ounce) package nonfat cream cheese, softened
- 1 cup nonfat sour cream
- 1 egg
- 3 egg whites
- ¼ cup cornstarch
- 1 tablespoon vanilla

Directions:

1. Preheat oven to 350°F. In medium bowl, combine gingersnap crumbs, walnuts, butter, and 2 tablespoons orange juice; mix until even. Press into bottom and up sides of 9″ springform pan; set aside in refrigerator.
2. In blender or food processor, combine cottage cheese, sugar, ¼ cup orange juice, and lemon juice; blend or process until very smooth. Scrape down sides and blend or process again.
3. In large mixing bowl, combine both packages of cream cheese and beat until smooth. Add sour cream; beat again until smooth. Add egg and beat well, then add cottage cheese mixture and beat well. Stir in egg whites, cornstarch, and vanilla and beat until smooth.
4. Pour cheese mixture into gingersnap crust. Bake for 50–60 minutes or until cheesecake is set around edges but still soft in center. Remove from oven and place on wire rack; let cool for 1 hour. Cover and refrigerate until cold, at least 4 hours.

Nutrition Info:

- Per Serving: Calories: 254.77; Fat: 9.11 g ;Saturated fat: 4.07 g;Sodium:206.98 mg

Peach Melba Frozen Yogurt Parfaits

Servings: 4

Cooking Time: 5 Minutes

Ingredients:

- 2 tablespoons slivered almonds
- 1 tablespoon brown sugar
- 2 peaches, peeled and chopped (see Ingredient Tip)
- 1 cup fresh raspberries
- 2 cups no-sugar-added vanilla frozen yogurt
- 2 tablespoons peach jam
- 2 tablespoons raspberry jam or preserves

Directions:

1. In a small nonstick skillet over medium heat, combine the almonds and brown sugar.
2. Cook, stirring frequently, until the sugar melts and coats the almonds, about 3 to 4 minutes. Remove from the heat and put the almonds on a plate to cool.
3. To make the parfaits: In four parfait or wine glasses, layer each with the peaches, raspberries, frozen yogurt, peach jam, and raspberry jam. Top each glass with the caramelized almonds.

Nutrition Info:

- Per Serving: Calories: 263 ; Fat: 5 g ;Saturated fat: 1 g ;Sodium: 91 mg

Apple Pear-nut Crisp

Servings: 8

Cooking Time: X

Ingredients:

- 2 apples, sliced
- 3 pears, sliced
- 2 tablespoons lemon juice
- ¼ cup sugar
- 1 teaspoon cinnamon
- ½ teaspoon nutmeg
- 1½ cups quick-cooking oatmeal
- ½ cup flour
- ¼ cup whole-wheat flour
- ½ cup brown sugar
- 1/3 cup butter or margarine, melted

Directions:

1. Preheat oven to 350ºF. Spray a 9″ round cake pan with nonstick cooking spray and set aside.
2. Prepare apples and pears, sprinkling with lemon juice as you work. Combine in medium bowl with sugar, cinnamon, and nutmeg. Spoon into prepared cake pan.
3. In same bowl, combine oatmeal, flour, whole-wheat flour, and brown sugar and mix well. Add melted butter and mix until crumbly. Sprinkle over fruit in dish.
4. Bake for 35–45 minutes or until fruit bubbles and topping is browned and crisp. Let cool for 15 minutes before serving.

Nutrition Info:

- Per Serving: Calories: 353.77; Fat:9.97 g ;Saturated fat: 5.25 g;Sodium: 61.78 mg

Double Chocolate Cinnamon Nice Cream

Servings: 4

Cooking Time: 5 Minutes

Ingredients:

- 3 tablespoons semisweet chocolate chips
- 2 frozen bananas, cut into chunks
- ⅓ cup frozen mango cubes
- 2 Medjool dates, pit removed and chopped (see Ingredient Tip)
- 2 tablespoons flax or soy milk
- 3 tablespoons cocoa powder
- ½ teaspoon vanilla extract
- ½ teaspoon ground cinnamon
- Pinch salt

Directions:

1. In a small saucepan over low heat, melt the semisweet chocolate chips, stirring frequently. Transfer the melted chocolate from the pan to a small bowl to cool, and place it in the refrigerator while you prepare the rest of the ingredients. (Make sure to not let the chocolate harden.)
2. In a blender or food processor, combine the bananas, mangoes, dates, and milk and blend until well combined.
3. Add the cocoa powder, vanilla, cinnamon, salt, and the melted, cooled chocolate. Blend until the mixture is smooth.
4. This treat can be served right away or frozen for 2 to 3 hours before serving.

Nutrition Info:

- Per Serving: Calories: 221 ; Fat: 5 g ;Saturated fat: 4 g ;Sodium: 8 mg

Mango Cheesecakes

Servings: X

Cooking Time: 35 Minutes

Ingredients:

- For the crust
- ¼ cup graham cracker crumbs
- 1 teaspoon avocado oil
- For the filling
- 4 ounces nonfat cream cheese, at room temperature
- ⅓ cup nonfat vanilla Greek yogurt, at room temperature
- 1 large egg
- ⅓ cup mango purée
- 2 tablespoons granulated sugar
- ½ teaspoon pure vanilla extract

Directions:

1. To make the crust
2. Preheat the oven to 300°F.
3. In a small bowl, toss together the crumbs and oil until combined. Evenly divide the mixture between 2 (6- to 8-ounce) ramekins. Press the crust into a thin layer in the bottom of each ramekin.
4. Place the ramekins in the oven and bake for 5 minutes. Remove from the oven and set aside.
5. To make the filling
6. In a medium bowl, beat the cream cheese on medium speed until very smooth, about 1 minute.
7. Add the yogurt and egg and continue beating until well blended. Scrape down the sides of the bowl and add the mango, sugar, and vanilla. Beat until completely smooth.
8. Spoon the filling into the ramekins and smooth the tops. Return them to the oven and bake until the centers are just set, about 30 minutes.
9. Cool the cheesecakes for 30 minutes on a wire rack, then transfer them to the refrigerator to chill completely, about 4 hours or overnight.
10. Serve.

Nutrition Info:

- Per Serving: Calories: 251 ; Fat: 7 g ;Saturated fat: 2 g ;Sodium: 98 mg

Pumpkin Pie Fruit Leathers

Servings: 10

Cooking Time: 8 Hours

Ingredients:

- 2 cups pumpkin purée
- 1 cup unsweetened applesauce
- 1 tablespoon maple syrup
- ¼ teaspoon ground cinnamon
- ⅛ teaspoon ground nutmeg
- ⅛ teaspoon ground ginger
- Pinch ground allspice

Directions:

1. Preheat the oven to the lowest setting possible or 150oF.
2. Line a baking sheet with parchment paper and set aside.
3. In a medium bowl, whisk together the pumpkin, applesauce, maple syrup, cinnamon, nutmeg, ginger, and allspice until very well blended. Spread the mixture on the baking sheet as evenly and thinly as possible.
4. Place the baking sheet in the oven and bake until the mixture is completely dried and no longer tacky to the touch, about 8 hours.
5. Remove the leather from the oven and cut into 10 pieces.

Nutrition Info:

- Per Serving: Calories: 33 ; Fat: 0 g ;Saturated fat: 0 g ;Sodium: 3 mg

Salted Caramel Pear And Blueberry Crisp

Servings: 4

Cooking Time: 20 Minutes

Ingredients:

- Nonstick cooking spray
- 2 pears, cored and chopped
- 1 cup fresh blueberries
- 2 tablespoons fresh lemon juice
- ¼ cup whole-wheat flour
- 2 tablespoons all-purpose flour
- ½ cup rolled oats
- 3 tablespoons packed brown sugar
- 1 teaspoon ground cinnamon
- 2 tablespoons butter, melted
- 2 tablespoons pear nectar or apple juice
- 2 tablespoons salted caramel sauce (see Ingredient Tip)

Directions:

1. Preheat the oven to 375°F. Spray the interiors of 4 (6-ounce) ramekins or custard cups with nonstick cooking spray and place on a cookie sheet. Set aside.
2. In a small bowl, combine the pears, blueberries, and lemon juice. Divide the mixture among the ramekins.
3. In a medium bowl, combine the whole-wheat flour, all-purpose flour, oats, brown sugar, and cinnamon, and mix well.
4. In a small bowl, combine the butter and pear nectar, and mix until smooth. Drizzle over the flour mixture and stir until crumbly.
5. Drizzle the caramel sauce over the fruit in each of the ramekins and top each with some of the oat mixture. Put the ramekins on a baking sheet to catch any drips.
6. Bake the crisps for 18 to 20 minutes or until they are golden brown on top and the fruit is bubbling.

Nutrition Info:

- Per Serving: Calories: 278 ; Fat: 7 g ;Saturated fat: 4 g ;Sodium: 59 mg

Whole-wheat Chocolate Chip Cookies

Servings: 48

Cooking Time: X

Ingredients:

- ¼ cup butter or plant sterol margarine, softened
- 1½ cups brown sugar
- ½ cup applesauce
- 1 tablespoon vanilla
- 1 egg
- 2 egg whites
- 2½ cups whole-wheat pastry flour
- ½ cup ground oatmeal
- 1 teaspoon baking soda
- ¼ teaspoon salt
- 2 cups special dark chocolate chips
- 1 cup chopped hazelnuts

Directions:

1. Preheat oven to 375°F. Line cookie sheets with parchment paper or Sil-pat silicone liners and set aside.
2. In large bowl, combine butter, brown sugar, and applesauce and beat well until smooth. Add vanilla, egg, and egg whites and beat until combined.
3. Add flour, oatmeal, baking soda, and salt and mix until a dough forms. Fold in chocolate chips and hazelnuts.
4. Drop dough by rounded teaspoons onto prepared cookie sheets. Bake for 7–10 minutes or until cookies are light golden brown and set. Let cool for 5 minutes before removing from cookie sheet to wire rack to cool.

Nutrition Info:

- Per Serving: Calories: 114.86; Fat:4.89 g ;Saturated fat:2.04 g;Sodium:26.49 mg

Dark Chocolate Meringues

Servings: 18

Cooking Time: 15 Minutes

Ingredients:

- 2 egg whites, at room temperature
- ⅓ cup granulated sugar
- 3 tablespoons confectioner's sugar
- ¼ cup cocoa powder
- Pinch salt
- ½ teaspoon vanilla extract
- ¼ cup mini semisweet chocolate chips

Directions:

1. Preheat the oven to 350°F. Line a baking sheet with parchment paper and set aside.
2. In a clean, dry medium bowl, place the egg whites. Put the bowl inside a larger bowl filled with very warm water and let stand for 5 minutes to warm up the egg whites.
3. Remove the medium bowl from the large bowl and carefully dry the outside.
4. In another medium bowl, sift together the granulated sugar, powdered sugar, cocoa powder, and salt.
5. Start beating the egg whites and gradually add the sugar mixture, beating constantly, until the mixture stands in peaks that droop when you pull up the turned-off beater.
6. Fold in the vanilla extract and the chocolate chips.
7. Drop by tablespoons onto the prepared baking sheet.
8. Bake for 13 to 15 minutes or until the meringues are set. Cool on the baking sheet for 5 minutes, then remove to a wire rack to completely cool. Store in layers separated by wax paper in an airtight container at room temperature up to 3 days.

Nutrition Info:

- Per Serving: Calories: 35 ; Fat: 1 g ;Saturated fat: 1 g

;Sodium: 9 mg

Lemon Mousse

Servings: 4

Cooking Time: X

Ingredients:

- 1 (0.25-ounce) envelope unflavored gelatin
- ¼ cup cold water
- 1/3 cup lemon juice
- 2/3 cup pear nectar
- ¼ cup sugar, divided
- 1 teaspoon grated lemon zest
- 1 cup lemon yogurt
- 2 pasteurized egg whites
- ¼ teaspoon cream of tartar

Directions:

1. In microwave-safe glass measuring cup, combine gelatin and cold water; let stand for 5 minutes to soften gelatin. Stir in lemon juice, pear nectar, and 2 tablespoons sugar. Microwave on high for 1–2 minutes, stirring twice during cooking time, until sugar and gelatin completely dissolve; stir in lemon zest. Let cool for 30 minutes.
2. When gelatin mixture is cool to the touch, blend in the lemon yogurt. Then, in medium bowl, combine egg whites with cream of tartar; beat until soft peaks form. Gradually stir in remaining 2 tablespoons sugar, beating until stiff peaks form.
3. Fold gelatin mixture into egg whites until combined. Pour into serving glasses or goblets, cover, and chill until firm, about 4–6 hours.

Nutrition Info:

- Per Serving: Calories: 151.27; Fat: 0.65 g ;Saturated fat: 0.40 g;Sodium:65.70 mg

Strawberry-rhubarb Parfait

Servings: 6

Cooking Time: X

Ingredients:

- 2 stalks rhubarb, sliced
- ½ cup apple juice
- 1/3 cup sugar
- 1 (10-ounce) package frozen strawberries
- 3 cups frozen vanilla yogurt

Directions:

1. In medium saucepan, combine rhubarb, apple juice, and sugar. Bring to a simmer, then reduce heat and simmer for 8–10 minutes or until rhubarb is soft.
2. Remove pan from heat and immediately stir in frozen strawberries, stirring to break up strawberries. Let stand until cool, about 30 minutes.
3. Layer rhubarb mixture and frozen yogurt in parfait glasses or goblets, starting and ending with rhubarb mixture. Cover and freeze until firm, about 8 hours.

Nutrition Info:

- Per Serving: Calories:210.56; Fat: 4.16 g ;Saturated fat: 2.48 g;Sodium: 64.41 mg

Chocolate Mousse Banana Meringue Pie

Servings: 8

Cooking Time: X

Ingredients:

- 1 recipe meringue pie shell
- 3 tablespoons cocoa powder
- 1 recipe Silken Chocolate Mousse
- 2 bananas, sliced
- 1 tablespoon lemon juice

Directions:

1. Follow directions to make meringue pie shell, but also beat cocoa into egg whites along with the sugar. Bake as directed in recipe. Let cool completely.
2. Make mousse as directed and chill in bowl for 4–6 hours until firm. Slice bananas, sprinkling lemon juice over slices as you work.
3. Layer mousse and sliced bananas in pie shell, beginning and ending with mousse. Cover and chill for 2–3 hours before serving.

Nutrition Info:

- Per Serving: Calories: 253.53; Fat:9.23 g ;Saturated fat: 5.94 g;Sodium:79.66 mg

Chocolate, Peanut Butter, And Banana Ice Cream

Servings: 2

Cooking Time: X

Ingredients:

- 2 frozen bananas, peeled and sliced
- 2 tablespoons cocoa powder
- 1 tablespoon honey
- 2 tablespoons all-natural peanut butter
- 1 tablespoon chopped walnuts (or nut of choice)

Directions:

1. Put the frozen bananas, cocoa powder, honey, and peanut butter into a high-speed blender and blend until smooth.
2. Transfer the ice cream mixture into a resealable container and freeze for 2 hours.
3. Once frozen, scoop the ice cream into two serving bowls and top with walnuts.

Nutrition Info:

- Per Serving: Calories: 269 ; Fat: 12 g ;Saturated fat: 2 g ;Sodium: 5 mg

Curried Fruit Compote

Servings: 6

Cooking Time: 10 Minutes

Ingredients:

- 1 (8-ounce) can pineapple chunks, undrained
- 1 ripe pear, peeled and chopped
- 1 Granny Smith apple, chopped
- ⅓ cup dried cranberries
- 1 cup apple juice
- 1 tablespoon fresh lemon juice
- 2 tablespoons agave nectar or packed brown sugar
- 1 tablespoon curry powder
- 1 tablespoon cornstarch
- Pinch salt

Directions:

1. In a medium saucepan over medium heat, combine the pineapple chunks, pear, apple, cranberries, apple juice, lemon juice, agave nectar (or brown sugar), curry powder, cornstarch, and salt. Stir to blend.
2. Bring to a boil, reduce the heat to low, and simmer for 6 to 8 minutes or until the fruit is tender.
3. At this point, you can serve the compote as-is, or you can purée all—or part—of it. The compote can be stored in the refrigerator for up to 3 days. You can re-warm the compote on the stovetop before you serve it.

Nutrition Info:

- Per Serving: Calories: 112 ; Fat: 0 g ;Saturated fat: 0 g ;Sodium: 4 mg

Chocolate-butterscotch Parfaits

Servings: 6

Cooking Time: X

Ingredients:

- 1 recipe Silken Chocolate Mousse
- 10 Butterscotch Meringues

- 6 tablespoons chopped hazelnuts, toasted
- 6 tablespoons butterscotch ice cream topping

Directions:

1. Prepare Silken Chocolate Mousse and refrigerate for 2 hours, until set. Prepare Butterscotch Meringues and let cool completely.
2. Break up meringues with your fingers. In six large parfait glasses, layer mousse and meringue crumbs, ending with the mousse. Sprinkle with toasted hazelnuts, cover, and chill for 2–4 hours.
3. Drizzle each parfait with 1 tablespoon butterscotch ice cream topping just before serving.

Nutrition Info:

- Per Serving: Calories: 365.51; Fat: 16.62 g ;Saturated fat: 8.27 g;Sodium: 179.64 mg

Green Grapes With Lemon Sorbet

Servings: 4

Cooking Time: X

Ingredients:

- 2 cups green grapes
- 2 tablespoons sugar
- ½ cup sweet white wine
- 1 teaspoon orange zest
- 2 cups lemon sorbet

Directions:

1. Wash grapes, dry, and cut in half. Sprinkle sugar over grapes and let stand for 5 minutes. Then add wine, stirring gently until sugar dissolves. Sprinkle with orange zest, cover, and refrigerate for 1 hour.
2. When ready to serve, stir grape mixture and serve over sorbet in sherbet glasses or goblets.

Nutrition Info:

- Per Serving: Calories: 233.90; Fat:1.61 g ;Saturated fat: 0.90 g;Sodium: 35.64 mg

Loaded Soy Yogurt Bowls

Servings: X

Cooking Time: X

Ingredients:

- 2 cups unsweetened vanilla soy yogurt
- 1 banana, sliced
- ½ cup raspberries or blueberries
- ¼ cup chopped pistachios
- ¼ cup roasted unsalted sunflower seeds
- 2 tablespoons honey
- 1 tablespoon hemp hearts, for garnish
- 1 tablespoon cacao nibs, for garnish

Directions:

1. Divide the yogurt between two bowls.
2. Evenly divide the banana, berries, pistachios, and sunflower seeds between the bowls.
3. Drizzle each bowl with 1 tablespoon of honey and top them with hemp hearts and cacao nibs.
4. Serve.

Nutrition Info:

- Per Serving: Calories: 394 ; Fat: 18 g ;Saturated fat: 2 g ;Sodium: 57 mg

Fruit Yoghurt Parfait

Servings: 2

Cooking Time: 20 Min

Ingredients:

- 2 cups plain Greek yogurt
- 1 banana, sliced
- ½ cup strawberries, sliced
- ¼ cup almonds, chopped
- ¼ cup unsalted sunflower seeds, roasted
- 2 tbsp. organic honey
- 1 tbsp. chia seeds, for garnish
- 1 tbsp. small dark chocolate chips, for garnish

Directions:

1. Divide the yoghurt between two serving bowls.
2. Evenly divide the banana, strawberries, almonds, and roasted sunflower seeds between the bowls.
3. Drizzle each bowl with 1 tbsp. of honey and top them with chia seeds and chocolate chips.
4. Serve cold.

Nutrition Info:

- Per Serving: Calories: 394 ; Fat: 18 g ;Saturated fat: 2 g ;Sodium: 57 mg

Chocolate Granola Pie

Servings: 12

Cooking Time: X

Ingredients:

- 3 tablespoons butter or margarine
- 2 (1-ounce) squares unsweetened chocolate, chopped
- ¼ cup brown sugar
- ½ cup dark corn syrup
- 2 teaspoons vanilla
- 1 egg
- 3 egg whites
- 2 cups Cinnamon Granola
- 1 Loco Pie Crust , unbaked

Directions:

1. Preheat oven to 350°F. In large saucepan, combine butter and chocolate. Melt over low heat, stirring frequently, until smooth. Remove from heat and add brown sugar, corn syrup, vanilla, egg, and egg whites and beat well until blended.
2. Stir in granola and pour into pie crust. Bake for 40–50 minutes or until filling is set and pie crust is deep golden brown. Let cool completely and serve.

Nutrition Info:

- Per Serving: Calories: 384.56; Fat:14.45 g ;Saturated fat:4.65 g;Sodium:137.51 mg

Fresh Peach Pie

Servings: 8

Cooking Time: X

Ingredients:

- 1½ cups graham-cracker crumbs
- 1/3 cup finely chopped walnuts
- 3 tablespoons canola oil
- 2 tablespoons butter or margarine, melted
- 1 (8-ounce) package light cream cheese, softened
- 1 cup powdered sugar
- 1 tablespoon vanilla
- 3 peaches
- 2 tablespoons lemon juice
- 1 cup Cinnamon Granola
- 1/3 cup toasted coconut

Directions:

1. In medium bowl, combine cracker crumbs and walnuts and mix well. Add oil and melted butter; stir with fork until crumbly. Press into bottom and up sides of 9″ pie pan; place in refrigerator.
2. In medium bowl, combine cream cheese with powdered sugar and vanilla; beat until light and fluffy. Spoon into bottom of pie crust; spread evenly.
3. Peel peaches and slice; sprinkle with lemon juice. Arrange over cream cheese filling in pie crust. Top with granola and coconut; cover and chill for at least 4 hours before serving.

Nutrition Info:

- Per Serving: Calories:294.10; Fat: 16.41 g ;Saturated fat: 5.45 g;Sodium: 186.80 mg

Almond Cheesecake–stuffed Apples

Servings: X

Cooking Time: 25 Minutes

Ingredients:

- 2 small apples, cut in half and cores scooped out on each side
- 1 teaspoon canola oil
- 2 tablespoons brown sugar, divided
- ⅛ teaspoon ground cinnamon
- ¼ cup fat-free cream cheese
- ⅛ teaspoon almond extract
- 2 tablespoons chopped almonds, for garnish

Directions:

1. Preheat the oven to 400°F.
2. Line a small baking dish with parchment paper and arrange the apple halves in the dish, cut-side up.
3. Brush the cut side of the apples with the canola oil. Sprinkle 1 tablespoon brown sugar and the cinnamon over the halves.
4. Place in the oven and bake for 15 minutes.
5. While the apples are baking, in a small bowl, stir together the cream cheese, remaining 1 tablespoon brown sugar, and almond extract until well blended.
6. Evenly divide the cream cheese mixture among the apple halves and bake for 10 more minutes.
7. Top with almonds and serve.

Nutrition Info:

- Per Serving: Calories: 307 ; Fat: 16 g ;Saturated fat: 7 g ;Sodium: 90 mg

30-Day Meal Plan

DAY	Breakfast	Lunch	Dinner
1	Pineapple Mixed Berry Smoothie 12	Creamy Vegetable Soup 22	Curried Garbanzo Beans 32
2	Tangy Fish And Tofu Soup 23	Panzanella Breakfast Casserole 12	Dark Beer Beef Chili 45
3	Blueberry Smoothie Bowl 13	Corn-and-chili Pancakes 34	Orange Thyme Red Snapper 67
4	Simple Pork Burgers 44	Apple Pear-nut Crisp 86	Fish Tacos 13
5	Pb&j Smoothies 13	Pork Cutlets With Fennel And Kale 45	Tofu And Root Vegetable Curry 33
6	Fresh Creamy Fruit Dip 23	Dutch Baby Pancakes 15	Seared Scallops With Fruit 66
7	Chopped Vegetable Tabbouleh 42	Tofu Scramble With Tomato And Spinach 16	Corn Polenta Chowder 26
8	Honey-garlic Sauce 82	Classic Italian Tomato Sauce 78	Spinach-ricotta Omelet 36
9	Spicy Butter Beans 25	Sour-cream-and-herb Omelet 40	Seaweed Rice Rolls 17
10	Peach Melba Frozen Yogurt Parfaits 85	Roasted Garlic Soufflé 41	Spinach Artichoke Pizza 18
11	Stuffed Mushrooms 37	Sweet Garlic-vinegar Crushed Cucumber 29	Fried Mahi-mahi 74
12	Oregano-thyme Sauce 77	Pepper Pot 49	Chicken Pesto 64
13	Chicken Pesto Baguette 20	Fresh Yellow-tomato Soup 28	Pumpkin And Chickpea Patties 35
14	Blueberry Almond Breakfast Bowl 20	Mustard Pork Tenderloin 50	Greek Quesadillas 26
15	Garbanzo Sandwich 38	Stir-fried Crispy Orange Beef 46	Spring Asparagus Soup 27

Low Cholesterol
Cookbook

DAY	Breakfast	Lunch	Dinner
16	Garbanzo Sandwich 41	Spicy Lentil Chili 24	Portobello Burgers 34
17	Lemon-cilantro Vinaigrette 78	German Potato Soup 25	Cod And Potatoes 75
18	Tomatoes With Chicken Mousse 64	Garbanzo Bean Salad 27	Lemon Garlic Flank Steak Wraps 47
19	Buttermilk Dressing 29	Pork Skewers With Cherry Tomatoes 46	Stuffed Noodle Squash 37
20	Strawberry-rhubarb Parfait 90	Smoky Barbecue Rub	Risotto With Artichokes 35
21	Peanut-butter-banana Skewered Sammies 42	Fruit-stuffed Pork Tenderloin 47	Smoky Bean And Lentil Chili 39
22	Mustard Berry Vinaigrette 81	Honey-garlic Chicken Stew 29	Pork Goulash 49
23	Buttermilk-herb Dressing 82	Pinto Bean Tortillas 40	Citrus Cod Bake 68
24	Green Grapes With Lemon Sorbet 91	Filet Mignon With Vegetables 53	Hawaiian Chicken Stir-fry 57
25	Simple Dijon And Honey Vinaigrette 79	Garbanzo Bean Pops 30	Cod Satay 70
26	Turkey Breast With Dried Fruit 60	Tzatziki 83	Navajo Chili Bread 19
27	Loaded Soy Yogurt Bowls 92	Italian Chicken Bake 58	Halibut Parcels 70
28	Spinach And Walnut Pesto 78	Rice-and-vegetable Casserole 39	Asian Chicken Stir-fry 59
29	Avocado Dressing 79	Double Chocolate Cinnamon Nice Cream 86	Thai Chicken Soup 22
30	Sweet Salad Dressing 77	Turkey Oat Patties 55	Seafood Risotto 71

Measurement Conversions

BASIC KITCHEN CONVERSIONS & EQUIVALENT

DRY MEASUREMENTS CONVERSION CHART

3 TEASPOONS = 1 TABLESPOON = 1/16 CUP

6 TEASPOONS = 2 TABLESPOONS = 1/8 CUP

12 TEASPOONS = 4 TABLESPOONS = 1/4 CUP

24 TEASPOONS = 8 TABLESPOONS = 1/2 CUP

36 TEASPOONS = 12 TABLESPOONS = 3/4 CUP

48 TEASPOONS = 16 TABLESPOONS = 1 CUP

METRIC TO US COOKING CONVER SIONS

OVEN TEMPERATURE

120℃ = 250° F

160℃ = 320° F

180℃ = 350° F

205℃ = 400° F

220℃ = 425° F

OVEN TEMPERATURE

8 FLUID OUNCES = 1 CUP = 1/2 PINT = 1/4 QUART

16 FLUID OUNCES = 2 CUPS = 1 PINT = 1/2 QUART

32 FLUID OUNCES = 4 CUPS = 2 PINTS = 1 QUART = 1/4 GALLON

128 FLUID OUNCES = 16 CUPS = 8 PINTS = 4 QUARTS = 1 GALLON

BAKING IN GRAMS

1 CUP FLOUR = 140 GRAMS

1 CUP SUGAR = 150 GRAMS

1 CUP POWDERED SUGAR = 160 GRAMS

1 CUP HEAVY CREAM = 235 GRAMS

VOLUME

1 MILLILITER = 1/5 TEASPOON

5 ML = 1 TEASPOON

15 ML = 1 TABLESPOON

240 ML = 1 CUP OR 8 FLUID OUNCES

1 LITER = 34 FL. OUNCES

WEIGHT

1 GRAM = .035 OUNCES

100 GRAMS = 3.5 OUNCES

500 GRAMS = 1.1 POUNDS

1 KILOGRAM = 35 OUNCES

US TO METRIC COOKING CONVERSIONS

1/5 TSP = 1 ML

1 TSP = 5 ML

1 TBSP = 15 ML

1 FL OUNCE = 30 ML

1 CUP = 237 ML

1 PINT (2 CUPS) = 473 ML

1 QUART (4 CUPS) = .95 LITER

1 GALLON (16 CUPS) = 3.8 LITERS

1 OZ = 28 GRAMS

1 POUND = 454 GRAMS

BUTTER

1 CUP BUTTER = 2 STICKS = 8 OUNCES = 230 GRAMS = 8 TABLESPOONS

BUTTER

1 CUP = 8 FLUID OUNCES

1 CUP = 16 TABLESPOONS

1 CUP = 48 TEASPOONS

1 CUP = 1/2 PINT

1 CUP = 1/4 QUART

1 CUP = 1/16 GALLON

1 CUP = 240 ML

BAKING PAN CONVERSIONS

1 CUP ALL-PURPOSE FLOUR = 4.5 OZ

1 CUP ROLLED OATS = 3 OZ 1 LARGE EGG = 1.7 OZ

1 CUP BUTTER = 8 OZ

1 CUP MILK = 8 OZ

1 CUP HEAVY CREAM = 8.4 OZ

1 CUP GRANULATED SUGAR = 7.1 OZ

1 CUP PACKED BROWN SUGAR = 7.75 OZ

1 CUP VEGETABLE OIL = 7.7 OZ

1 CUP UNSIFTED POWDERED SUGAR = 4.4 OZ

BAKING PAN CONVERSIONS

9-INCH ROUND CAKE PAN = 12 CUPS

10-INCH TUBE PAN =16 CUPS

11-INCH BUNDT PAN = 12 CUPS

9-INCH SPRINGFORM PAN = 10 CUPS

9 X 5 INCH LOAF PAN = 8 CUPS

9-INCH SQUARE PAN = 8 CUPS

Date: _____

MY SHOPPING LIST

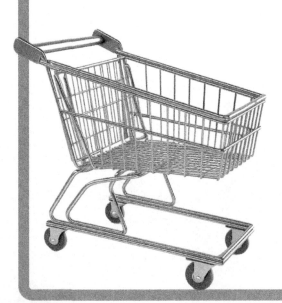

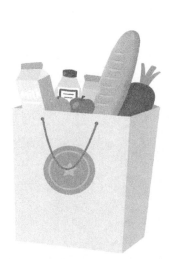

Recipe ....

From the kicthen of ....

Serves .... Prep time .... Cook time ....

☐ Difficulty   ☐ Easy   ☐ Medium   ☐ Hard

Ingredient   *Yummy!*

....

....

....

....

....

Directions ....

....

....

....

....

....

....

Recipe for:

Ingredients:

Equipment:

Description:

Instructions:

Low Cholesterol
Cookbook

Appendix : Recipes Index

Printed in Great Britain
by Amazon

41053637R00057